Andre

VACCINE FREE

111 Stories of Unvaccinated Children

Illustrated by
Alena Ryazanova
(ralena2005@gmail.com)

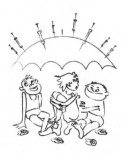

This book is not intended to provide any medical advice or to replace the treatment of a physician. The decision on whether to vaccinate your children or yourself is entirely left up to you. I hope the information given in this book will help you to make an informed decision.

Published by Andreas Bachmair

Copyright © 2012 Andreas Bachmair
www.vaccineinjury.info
www.vaccinefree.info
All rights reserved.

ISBN-10: 1478396520
EAN-13: 9781478396529

Content

Acknowledgments v
Forewords vii
    I vii
    II viii
    III x
    IV xi
Introduction 1
Stories of unvaccinated children 7
    USA 7
    Canada 85
    UK 105
    Australia 119
    New Zealand 127
    Norway 131
    Iceland 133
    Poland 135
    Netherlands 137
    Germany 139
    United Arab Emirates 143
    Indonesia 145
    India 147
Appendix 149
New Children Book! 157

Acknowledgments

I wish to thank all the gracious participants in the survey on the state of health of unvaccinated children and in particular the families who were willing to share their stories in this book.

I thank Alena Ryazanova for her beautifully expressive illustrations and the fun I had working with her.

I thank Dr. James Bowman, MD, ND, for proofreading and editing the book and his valuable feedback given to me throughout this time.

I thank Betsy Mayer for translating and editing the German stories into English. I also want to thank her for the translation of the German website www.impfschaden.info into English, because without the English website www.vaccineinjury.info this book would have never come into being.

I thank Andreas Ruttkamp for his on-going technical support of my website and the implementation of my (sometimes "creative") ideas.

I thank Sebastian Lentz for his advice and wonderful suggestions.

I thank Dr. Sherri Tenpenny for her continued support of my survey, and posting many calls for participation on her Facebook page.

I thank everyone who wrote me wonderful emails supporting my work and my ongoing effort to bring the truth to the people.

And last but not least I want to thank my family for their love and support I received in bringing forth this book.

Andreas Bachmair
September 24th, 2012

Forewords

I

Andreas Bachmair and I met seemingly by accident some years ago, but in reflecting upon that meeting, it now seems anything but accidental. I believe, rather, that it was my great good fortune and destiny to meet him as I find him a rare and fascinating combination of very practical and common sense knowledge tempered with a high degree of solid, scientific understanding of the complexities and subtleties of human biology. I have known many practitioners during my career in medicine, and he is a most rare find, a man of intelligence, integrity, humility and courage, and someone I could not respect or admire more than I do. I strongly recommend this book, knowing that the time you spend reading it will be time well spent, an investment in yourself and your children, which will indeed bring many rewards to your future health.

James R. Bowman, MD, ND, DNHC, DCP, FAAIM, DiHom

Biography

Dr. James R. Bowman took his training in medicine and homeopathy in Europe because the best academic training and education in biology and science is found in Europe. He has been in daily clinical family practice for over 35 years and although trained at first in classical allopathic medicine, soon found it to be extremely lacking in logic or results. Because of this, like Dr. Samuel Hahnemann, MD, the discoverer and founder of homeopathy, he began to study other options, and based on those scientific facts and the outcome for patients, he has devoted his work exclusively to natural and alternative medicine for decades. He has a small, private family clinic in the United States (Wisconsin) and works with both children and adults for a very wide variety of health issues, using strictly natural and alternative methods. If you would like to learn more about his work please visit his website: www.getyourlifeback.org

---

II

Vaccine Free – 111 Stories of Unvaccinated Children is a very moving testament to the power of the body to take care of itself and the trust that people put in that natural process.

As a species, we humans have come to distrust our bodies, distrust our ability to read the signs that our bodies are telling us and to place all that displaced trust in a system of medicine that is merely 100 years old.

The wisdom of centuries old herbal, nutritional and energy medicine has been swept aside in the rush to embrace science-based medicine.

In my private practice that I began in 1979 I made the decision to offer homeopathic alternatives to mercury-based vaccinations. I simply felt that I was following the Hippocratic Oath "First Do No Harm." I can only assume that the medical community ignores the obvious damage done by mercury because they don't want to admit the harm they inflict on their patients.

In a soon-to-be-published book, *Mercury Mayhem*, I outline "The Downward Spiral of Mercury Toxicity." This descent into a life of illness explains why some parents make the decision to not vaccinate their children. These 21 points are a composite story of a mother and a child who follow the mainstream protocols and do what they are told by their doctors. But you should know that in medical school doctors are not even told about the use of mercury in medicine or dentistry. Doctors are never warned about its dangers.

Since toxicity caused by mercury is not a topic of study in medical school, most doctors are not aware of the spiral of illness that it causes. In my medical school, I was told that if I didn't learn something in my medical training, then it didn't exist, or it was just plain quackery. This arrogant stance has left many patients feeling completely hopeless in the grip of brain-numbing mercury toxicity.

Of course there are other poisons in vaccinations that only add to the toxic soup that is shot into helpless children in a way that's completely alien. My point is that kids only get ill when they are already run down, malnourished and stressed emotionally or physically. When those criteria are met, germs that normally inhabit our environment find their way into a receptive body through air, food or water. So, the very "germ theory" on which vaccinations are based, is erroneous.

If you want to be inspired to take your power into your own hands, read this book to keep your children safe and well.

Thanks and high praise to Andreas Bachmair for producing this wonderful book. And to the many thousands of parents who are brave enough and wise enough to do what it takes to keep their children safe. To me, these parents are heroes and deserve our highest regard.

Dr. Carolyn Dean

Biography

Dr. Carolyn Dean is a medical doctor and naturopathic doctor in the forefront of the natural medicine revolution since 1979. She is the author/coauthor of 28 health books (print and eBooks) including Death by Modern Medicine, Future Health Now Encyclopedia, The Magnesium Miracle, Kids Health: A Doctor's Guide for Parents, Homeopathic Remedies for Children's Common Ailments, IBS for Dummies, IBS Cookbook for Dummies, The Yeast Connection and Women's Health, Everything Alzheimer's, and Hormone Balance. Dr. Dean is the Medical Director of the non-profit educational site - Nutritional Magnesium Association, www.nutritionalmagnesium.org. She has a free online newsletter and a valuable online 2-year wellness program called Completement Now! She also runs a busy telephone consulting practice. www.drcarolyndean.com.

III

For quite some time, many parents who have started to do their own research into the safety and efficacy of vaccines being pushed on their children have been asking the question "Why have there been no studies comparing vaccinated to unvaccinated children?" This is a very important question as increasing numbers of parents are watching their children receive increasing numbers of vaccines, accompanied by increasing incidence of allergies, anaphylactic shock, autism and other neurological conditions, all autoimmune diseases, and cancer. Is it not self evident that any claim that vaccines are not behind this epidemic of immune system diseases would have to start with just such a comparison?

As the vaccine promoters who are funded by Big Pharma continue to deny the self evident fact that the increase in the childhood vaccine schedule directly parallels the increase in autoimmune disease and cancer, parents are finally checking things out for themselves instead of beLIEving the denials of the white coated "experts". When a normal 15 month old child receives the MMR vaccine and shortly thereafter loses eye contact and speech, starts flapping their hands and doing other unusual behaviors, their pediatricians always deny the obvious correlation. They will usually blame the genes of the parents (even when there has never been any history of the disorder in either family). They will claim that numerous studies (always funded by Big Pharma) have never shown any correlation of vaccines with disease of the immune system.

In reality, the most important part of the scientific method is OBSERVATION. If you stub your toe on a rock and it subsequently becomes swollen and turns blue, there is an obvious cause and effect relationship. However, when the temporal relationship of a vaccine assault with subsequent injury is reported, the vaccinator will without fail always claim that the injury could NOT be due to vaccines. Why is this denial occurring, making vaccines the "sacred cow" of medicine? Is there a fear that the millions of lives that have been destroyed by this insane practice of vaccination would lead to a global outcry the likes of which has never been seen in history? How could people ever trust medical doctors again? And without Big Pharma controlled medical doctors to prescribe their toxic poisons (when there are natural solutions for all diseases already available), how could the Big Pharma companies stay in business? THEY COULD NOT. As the author states in his introduction, FOLLOW THE MONEY.

The study done by Andreas Bachmair and reported in this very important book and the personal stories of unvaccinated children reveal the tremendous difference in immune system disease between unvaccinated and vaccinated children. Even more importantly, he has validated what I have realized after 15 years of teaching people how to reverse their vaccine induced diseases (which encompass pretty much all of the diseases under "internal medicine"); that ALL OF THE UNVACCINATED CHILDREN WITH IMMUNE DYSFUNCTION WERE BORN OF VACCINATED PARENTS! What this proves is that the vaccine viruses injected into the parents can be transmitted to the fetus. I realized this after the handful of my clients with autism whose parents had not vaccinated them responded to my Hippocrates protocol (detoxing vaccine viruses with homeopathy) just as their vaccinated peers did. This tells us that the epidemic of VIDS (vaccine induced disease) will become worse with each vaccinated generation, which is why I have dedicated my life to putting an end to VIDS; the biggest epidemic the world has ever known! Please spread the word.

Rebecca Carley, MD

Rebecca Carley, MD, Court Qualified Expert in VIDS, Hickory, NC, USA
www.reversingvaccineinduceddiseases.com

IV

I was lucky to be brought up in a family where my father did not follow public opinion - especially in regards to my health. Although he started his professional career as a pharmacist he did not agree with what was happening in the drug industry back in the 1950's. He left pharmacy after 6 years in the field and became a chiropractor. In order for him to do this, he had to fly from New Zealand to the USA and study in Davenport Iowa.

My father was a very passionate chiropractor and 53 years later, he is still practicing at the age of 84. 52 years ago, the vaccine program in Australia was delivered in the school system, nobody questioned the program everyone did the same thing and followed the vaccine protocol and schedule. I remember being the only child left in the schoolroom during the routine vaccines as my father would not give permission for me to be vaccinated. At the time, I didn't really think too much about it, but many of the girls would say I was lucky because I didn't have to have a needle in my arm. A Chinese proverb says "A wise man does not follow public opinion he makes his own decisions", and I believe my dad was one of the wise men.

My dad not only would not give me or my siblings vaccines but he was also opposed to antibiotics for infections and pain killers for tooth eruptions. So at the age of 52 I have never had an antibiotic or any prescribed or non prescribed medication. Many doctors say I'm just lucky and so do many people but what they don't realize is that on the part of my father it was very good management of my health. My mother cooked everything from scratch as did many women in the 1960's and 1970's, we were encouraged to live an active lifestyle and I was under chiropractic care from the day I was born.

My family questioned public opinion and medical dogma and it is hard once you have been taught to do this not to continue it through out life.

When I became pregnant with my first child in 1988, I questioned everything. I didn't want any ultra sounds and I refused to swallow the flavored, colored, sugar laden glucose mixture for a pregnancy glucose tolerance test that was advised to see if I had gestational diabetes. When my son was born I would not let them give him vitamin K, the recommended vitamin for newborns due to the rise in hemorrhagic disease. I did not refuse these routine procedures lightly; I read all the current research.

Vaccinations were also something else that I looked into fully. I read everything I could. I had done immunology during my six years at university, but I wanted to see both sides of the story. My husband was not quite so sure, but decided that I knew more than he did and left the decision in my hands. A couple of years later he thanked me for my foresight and voracious need for knowledge to know that vaccines were safe (or not).

After all my reading on vaccines I actually became fearful of them, I was more scared for my children to have a vaccine than I was of the childhood disease it was meant to prevent. I also followed my fathers lead and would not give my children antibiotics. Of course if it was life threatening I would have given them what they needed. I also decided that the first pain my children would really feel was the pain of their teeth coming through their gums. I, like my parents,decided not to give my children any pain relief as I wanted their pain mechanisms to get some practice. I figured if they could deal with the small infections and small pains in life without drugs then their bodies' immune system and pain centers would be primed for the larger infections and pains they may experience as they grew and went out into the world.

Controversy and emotion are two words that can be said about the vaccination debate. Those that oppose it do it after much reading and consideration. Most people who vaccinate their children either do it because it is public policy, fear or they trust implicitly in the process. When I was asked to be in a survey to determine the health of unvaccinated and vaccinated children I jumped at the chance. I have my story but I wanted to know if other people had similar stories with their unvaccinated children.

I'm a speaker and a health advocate and after every talk I'm approached by quite a few people telling me about what happened to their child after a vaccination. Some were death, others autism or some neurological complaint. I didn't hear too many heart-breaking stories from parents who had not vaccinated.

I was sent an email from a friend who had heard of the research Andreas Bachmair was doing, she felt that myself and my adult children would be a wonderful addition to the research. I thought at last we have someone who is interested in the health of unvaccinated children. I always wondered why someone would not research a family as mine as we don't depend on the national social health system. I always felt that it would be better to research people who have health rather than to research people who have lost their health. Research is targeted for cure rather than for prevention. Until Andreas's research came along there was no one interested in families with health.

Andreas's research will be ongoing and in my way of thinking some of the most important research on vaccination effects and long-term health of those that are vaccinated and unvaccinated.

Albert Einstein said that those who have the privilege to know have the duty to act and Andreas's work will continue to educate people in order to know about vaccination and the long term effects. His research will educate people to not follow public opinion and propaganda but rather question what is happening and become informed when making decisions that pertain to the health of our future generations.

Cyndi O'Meara

Cyndi O'Meara, P.O. Box 104, Mooloolaba Q 4557, International Speaker, Best Selling Author, TV and Radio Presenter, www.changinghabits.com.au

Introduction

Since the introduction of vaccinations 200 years ago great controversy has surrounded them. Some people believe that certain illnesses are very dangerous and out of fear, rather than sound scientific knowledge, they react by seeing vaccines as a safe and effective way to avoid illness and possibly even eradicate them. If one reacts out of fear, rather than accurate, factual scientific knowledge, then one's actions will be directed by one's emotions, often resulting in negative, rather than positive, health outcomes for both parents and children.

If, on the other hand, one bases one's decisions on clear, proven, objective scientific truths, one's actions are not ruled by fear or other emotions, and often the outcomes are far more humane and positive for everyone involved. There is a rapidly growing movement of scientists, doctors, and parents who subscribe to this approach when dealing with the question of vaccinations.

Who could possibly be against such scientific truth and logic? There is an old phrase that has great meaning here: "Follow the money!" It means that whoever will benefit financially from a certain cultural and legislative phenomenon is the one to watch and to question because financial interests often pervert and undermine solid, proven scientific truths.

Who benefits from vaccines? The drug companies, no one else, except the politicians who can be influenced or bought by the extremely powerful financial resources of the drug companies. If it is the drug companies and the politicians who benefit, then who is it who does not? The families, the children and parents, they are the financial, political and biological victims, they suffer the loss, they are the ones who are damaged.

In Washington, DC, the capitol of the United States, there are 435 elected members of the Congress and 100 elected senators whose job it is to represent the best interests of the American people as they write legislation to protect citizens and defend their rights. Did you know that in Washington, DC there are more than 1500 paid lobbyists, working for the special interest groups like drug companies who constantly attempt to influence politicians to write legislation favorable to the profits of the drug companies at the expense, and sometimes the very lives, of American citizens?

It is true – there are three paid lobbyists for every single elected official in Washington. If it seems the deck is stacked against anyone holding a differing point of view, this is why. If you do not vaccinate your children then your pediatrician may refuse to work with you, and he or she may actually report you to the State Health Office as being negligent and abusive to your children because you have not vaccinated them.

DHHS (Department of Health & Human Services) administers these matters and frequently they will confront parents who have chosen not to vaccinate their children with threats of legal action, punishment, fines, and in some cases, threats of having the children taken from their parents because of non-compliance with the recommendations of the drug companies and the medical providers who represent and defend them.

Who controls all health care, all health care legislation, all medical training, research and education? The drug companies. They control the legislatures, the training of doctors and nurses, and all medical research. So instead of having a neutral, unbiased situation in which people are free do conduct their own research and make their own best informed decisions based on facts, those rights are taken from them with threats of punishment, fines and even losing their children because they chose to challenge a system of health care which demands parents expose their children to dozens of different toxic substances which science has proven do not work well, and which have serious and sometimes fatal side effects.

Human beings are born with innate protective systems called immune systems which are biologically designed to identify and neutralize any invading pathogenic organism, whether it is a bacterium or virus or parasite. Additionally our skin is both a physical barrier and a chemical barrier protecting us from invading organisms. There are chemicals and oils in our skin which protect us from such infections, and if the organisms do gain access to us internally, then the immune system mobilizes a huge and impressive series of reactions to quickly and effectively neutralize the threat. It seems only logical that we should work with our already existing biological defense system which has evolved over millions of years, finding safe, effective ways to enhance and strengthen it when necessary, rather than working against this wonderful, competent system by injecting toxic substances based on 100 years of drug company dominance in politics.

In the United States each state has three legal waivers which parents can choose if they oppose vaccinating their children. There are legally recognized waivers for personal reasons, medical reasons, and religious reasons, and parents have the legal right to challenge any demand from anyone that they must vaccinate their children, but many parents are either unaware of these rights, or they are frightened and intimidated by the extremely aggressive efforts of the DHHS and other public health authorities.

Beyond "Follow the money," there is another critical principle at play here: truth. The very last thing in the world the drug companies or all the people they control (the media, politicians, legislators, doctors, nurses, public health workers) want to happen is that you learn the truth – that is their greatest fear. If they keep you ignorant and reacting out of fear, then they have you right where they want you, under their thumb, completely believing their false and inaccurate philosophy instead of thinking for yourself, investigating for yourself, doing your own independent research and learning that vaccines are dangerous and do not work.

Whether you choose to vaccinate is and should solidly remain your own personal decision. Vaccination questions are complex, there are no easy black-and-white answers, every parent must deliberate carefully before deciding, but God has given these children to you for safekeeping, it is not only your right, but your sacred responsibility to protect them from any potential harm.

For this reason, loving and protecting your children has to be the first and the final criterion to consider when you are deciding about vaccinating your children. If you investigate this thoroughly and without prejudice you will find solid, credible scientific sources of information which give you both insight and understanding of the biological aspects of children's health, as well as empowerment to exercise your rights to be a strong, protective parent and have as your highest priority the safety and welfare of the children God has entrusted to your care.

In this book, based on my research with more than 14,000 participants from all over the world, you will find the stories of families who investigated these issues carefully and thoughtfully because they love and want to protect their children. If the true scientific evidence proved vaccines were safe and effective there would be no debate, no argument, and no controversy. The very fact that there is such widespread debate over this issue itself proves that what the drug companies claim and want you to believe is highly questionable and unreliable, something each thinking parents needs to investigate for themselves.

In this book you will read diverse thinking about children and vaccines. I wanted to present a broad range of views and opinions so all sides of the story would be considered. The stories are as the parents wrote them, I did not edit them in any way, I wanted to preserve the purity of each family's thoughts.

As everyone is unique, like their fingerprints and DNA, I wanted the uniqueness of each individual story to speak for itself. It is my sincere hope that in reading this book you will consider your role as a parent and protector of your children, that you will investigate the issues deeply, carefully, and thoughtfully, always putting the health and welfare of your children first, where it belongs.

Introduction

I, too, am a father, and in our family we have discussed this at great length. We did a lot of exhaustive research, asked a lot of probing and difficult questions, always with the aim of finding the truth and causing no harm to our family. I hope that in reading this book that will be your experience as well. Thank you.

Andreas Bachmair,
Family Homeopathic Practitioner
Switzerland

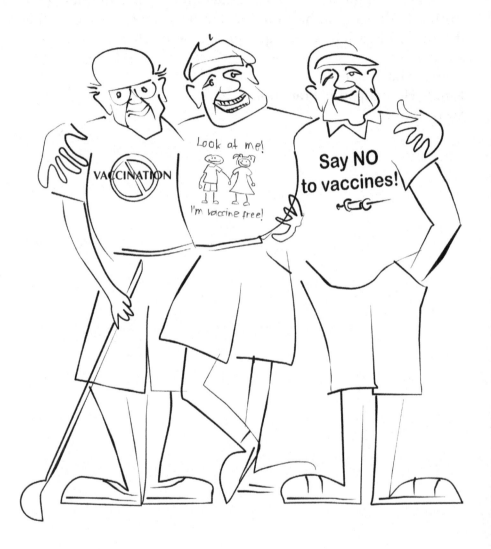

Stories of unvaccinated children

USA

"I am an unvaccinated child, 74 years of age. I have two brothers, aged 70 and 76, neither of whom was subjected to vaccination. None of us have had any serious disease or has spent time in a hospital. I have never had a flu shot or any other kind of shot. Good health is first of all a gift of God, but it is also greatly dependent on how we care for our bodies. Part of that care is insuring that there is no defilement of the blood stream."

"Savannah's story began 18 months ago. Savannah is a loving gift from God brought to us through adoption. She was born September 8, 2010 in San Antonio, TX. She was born to a mother taking several different psychiatric medications. I asked the birth mother if she would please not allow Savannah to receive the Hep. B vaccine after birth. She agreed with me, so I created a document stating she did not want her baby to receive the Hep. B and she gave this paper to her doctor. I was present in the hospital when the doctor asked why she did not want the Hep. B. The birth mother stood her ground and opposed the shot. I told the doctor that I was exercising my conscientious belief which TX has the Conscientious Exemption and the doctor quickly accepted my decision as the adoptive parent. Once we arrived home in Pensacola, FL, we went to the public health clinic and got the Religious Exemption. Which was extremely easy to do? We made sure to include a copy into our file for the agency conducting our post placement visits in FL. The agency in Texas accepted our decision believing it's every parent's right to choose.

Savannah was born with thrush. Her pediatrician who is an integrative/holistic pediatrician said it came from the birth mother because young women are so yeasty these days. I gave her some strong probiotics made for infants and she healed well. Savannah is an extremely bright little girl. She's eager to learn and picks up new things quickly. She has a memory like an elephant. She's extremely strong and can run very fast. She has been sick only a few times. She had diarrhea twice which both times she picked up from playing at Jamboree. She healed quickly and had no complications. She probably had Rotavirus because it was pretty bad and now she has natural immunity. She has had a cold 2 times in her entire 18 months of life. She had normal cold-like symptoms and healed quickly. She has never had an ear infection. Her scrapes and bruises heal very quickly, too. Savannah loves to communicate learning new words every day. She's very coordinated loving to kick balls and throw with accuracy. She's not afraid of the water. She loves her blanket and loves her family. She recognizes strangers. Her imagination is keen. She has named several of her dolls with names she chose. She seems so much more alert than a lot of her peers. Savannah is a stay at home baby and has never been in a daycare. She does go into the church nursery. I know in my heart we made the right decision to not vaccinate."

"My son has never been vaccinated. He is the youngest of five children and his older brothers and sister were vaccinated because I hadn't researched the issues with vaccines when they were born. I didn't realize there were problems with vaccines until my midwife mentioned the issue when I was pregnant with him. I had previously gone to obstetricians and had hospital births (His was also my best birth, but that's another story!). His siblings were frequently sick, especially with ear infections. He has NEVER had an ear infection. He has rarely been ill at all and has never been to a doctor. He is very calm, affectionate, and intelligent. He has never had any learning difficulties or hyperactivity problems. Since he has never been to a doctor I never had to deal with their pressure to vaccinate, but I used to lie awake at night worrying that somehow it would be found out and they would try to take him away from me. I also wondered if I was wrong somehow and he would get some horrible disease. Now he is 13 years old and none of my fears materialized."

"We have 2 children, one who is 6 and another who is almost 3. Our older child had a seizure within 20 minutes of having a DPT shot right around 6 months old. Although the pediatric Dr.'s refused to acknowledge the vaccine causing the seizure, we did halt all vaccines and will never vaccinate again. This frightening experience led to tons of reading and thinking things through, and also the choice to not vaccinate our second child. Both of our children are very healthy kids, compared to their friends and schoolmates. They don't catch the flu or pertussis or any of the other major illnesses highly vaccinated against yet so easily spread amongst the vaccinated. I am a firm believer in chiropractic health, and have seen how good spine health directly affects children's well being. I am also a firm believer that we as parents know the best choice for our kids, and that Big Pharma has no interest in them whatsoever. I am grateful for the good health of my children, and for the awesome alternative care out there!"

"I am a mother of 3 boys, all unvaccinated. I am also unvaccinated, as is my mother and hers. Since I spent my growing years hearing the adults discuss vaccination and listening to the sometimes difficult dealings with schools I was pretty aware of the family's choices. When I began having children I researched each disease and each vaccine. My husband and I chose not to vaccinate. I couldn't be more comfortable with our decision. Some of the diseases do scare me, but so do the vaccines. I just don't think you can get around being scared about the unknowable future, whichever way you go. In addition to not vaccinating, we choose a healthy lifestyle for our family (breast feeding as babies and mostly whole foods as children). We seek natural remedies when needed and chiropractic as well. Between all 3 boys (ages 7, 5, and 3 months) there have only been a few short lived (1-2 day) ear infections, no cases of the flu and one minor cough. The older boys have had chicken pox and I am thankful for it. As a child I had minor cases of chicken box, measles, rubella and mumps and I believe it has made me healthier. It has helped me pass on immunities to my children as well."

"I have two girls ages 14 and 11 who have never had a vaccination. This includes the hepatitis B they like to give newborns.

We made the decision not to vaccinate after much research. We believe in the body's ability to self-heal when given the proper nutrients, and in the body's inborn immune system when allowed to grow and function naturally.

We fed them differently than most and exclusively breastfed until they were 6 months adding in carrot juice. When they had teeth, 9 months for the first and 8 months for the second, we began feeding them apples. We added in other fruits slowly. Then we added sweet potatoes and avocados and finally other vegetables. They got starches once they had molars and they didn't taste sugar until they were 2. They did not eat jarred food, drink formula, milk or bottled juices. I say this because I feel that this diet along with no vaccines have given us amazingly healthy children.

Neither have had anything more serious than a cold and most of the time they are up and playing within 24 hours. We also do not treat fevers but let them run their course and do their job of killing germs. Neither girls have any cavities either, and do not use fluoride toothpaste or drink milk.

We do not use western medicine and are naturopathic when treating illness. My husband and I were both vaccinated and taken to doctors regularly. We have watched what happens when you step outside the traditional ways and look to nature and common sense for healing."

"I have 3 sons ages 7, 5, and 2 and they have never been vaccinated. We chose to simply delay the vaccinations when our first son was born but as he got older and we had more kids, we decided to delay indefinitely. They have been very healthy boys! They have never had ear infections or any of the "typical" childhood illnesses. They have each in turn had a bad cold when they were babies, but they are rarely sick now. And when they are (once in the last 9 months) it consists of feeling tired for a day or two and a stuffed nose for just as long. While we always choose natural remedies and wholesome food to strengthen their bodies, we fully believe by not vaccinating we have kept their immune systems working properly and healthy. In a world of antibiotics, our boys have never had a single dose! We homeschool our children which also helps them from being bombarded with daily germs but we are out and about town frequently and often come into contact with kids their age who are usually always suffering from runny noses or throwing up, especially during winter and spring.

My 7-year-old son has a pretty strong food intolerance to gluten and dairy. We discovered it when he was 3 after noticing severe digestion issues. My youngest son, almost 2, has an eczema reaction to eggs. Their food intolerances make me even more grateful that we didn't vaccinate. I have read and fully believe in the gut/brain connection. If their bodies had been given vaccines as newborns and followed the recommended schedule, I have no doubt that we would be seeing some serious psychological or neurological issues with it now. Instead, all we have to deal with is where to find good vegan food when we are out, and the very occasional cold. We are truly happy with our decision not to vaccinate!"

"I never received vaccinations nor did my child. I am a mother of 2 year-old-son and one on the way. My son has never gotten one shot in his life and is the healthiest child out of all the kids we do play group with! The others are always sick, allergies, runny noses etc. He has never made a trip to the doctor or needed it.

Both myself and my sister never received vaccinations as children or adults and both of us have outstanding health! I have been around people who have Chicken Pox and never caught it, also around others who were very sick and never caught their illnesses as well.

My son is off the charts with hand eye coordination, speaking ability and other 'milestones' kids reach at this point. We are very happy with our decision and will continue to back it up with organic eating, juicing and homeopathic remedies for anything that comes along."

"After my daughter, who is now 8 years old, suffered adverse reactions to her vaccinations, I decided to stop vaccinating her when she was a year and a half. I believe that her vaccines are responsible for her multiple food allergies, eczema, and asthma. After much research, I decided that I would not continue vaccinating her. My son was born in 2006 and has not had any vaccinations. Even though I felt that vaccinations were the cause of my daughter's issues, I was still scared NOT to vaccinate my son. I was always taught that vaccinations were safe and to not get them was at one time not an option for me. But, after careful consideration I felt that not vaccinating my children was probably the best thing for them. I went back and forth on this.

My daughter has improved much and my son is the healthiest kid I know. We live in a military community with many kids. I would say at least 90% of our housing has children of various ages. There is always some illness going around, whether it is a stomach bug or some respiratory issue. Most kids at the school miss several days of school a year due to an illness. My son has been going to daycare since the age of 18 months, starting in New Hampshire. He never missed a day of daycare due to illness. It was common for at least one or two kids to be out, especially during the winter months due to illness. He has never had to be seen by a doctor except for his physical/well-child check ups (for school), and once when he was 10 months old for oral thrush, which I blame my diet (I was breastfeeding at the time). He has never had an ear infection. He has vomited several times the past few years, but he vomits one time and he is over what it was that made him sick. If he ever has an elevated temp, I encourage fluids and rest, and he is over it the next day.

He now attends kindergarten at a public school. He has never missed a day of school, whereas my daughter has missed at least 5 days. He is always around children who are sick and rarely even has a runny nose. Lately, there was a cold that sent one little girl to the hospital for 2 weeks and she was diagnosed with RSV. The group of children and the adults my kids are around were all sick. My son also caught this, but he suffered mainly from a stuffy nose and was over it within a week. A week later, the other children were still fighting off this cold.

He has no allergies, no asthma, and no skin issues. He is a very happy and bright child. In New Hampshire, he would be in preschool, but California's cut off for entering kindergarten is later, so he was 4 when he first entered kindergarten. He is advanced in his reading and math. I believe that much of the issues that vaccinations cause not only affect a child's physical health, but also their mental health. My daughter, with all her allergies and eczema, is distracted by her discomfort and it has affected her school work.

The more I see how my son rarely ever has issues regarding his health, the more comfortable and pleased I am with the decision to not vaccinate. We still have to go to the doctor to have them do his physical/check-ups, where I do get an earful and they try to give me guilt-trips. "You would feel so bad if he caught a disease that was vaccine-preventable". I let it go in one ear and out the other because as bad as I would feel if he were to get sick, I would feel worse crippling his immune system to afford him that "protection". I've seen what it did to my daughter...and now she is living with lifelong issues. Why would I repeat the same mistake?"

"My daughter is 4 years old and has not had any vaccines. She is a beautiful and intelligent child. She is curious and very healthy. We live a normal life and she goes to preschool and is involved in all the same activities as other children her own age. She has been very healthy with only the occasional trip to the doctor. In fact we went a whole year without going to the doctor last year. She has only had two fevers and only the occasional mild cold. She does not suffer from any chronic problems.

Sometimes we do doubt our decision not to vaccinate but then when I think about injecting her with all the toxins in the vaccines I stop myself from doubting. She is pure and beautiful and her immune system functions perfectly. She has organic pure foods to eat and gets good sleep; in fact we have never had any problems with sleep. I breast-fed her until she was 12 months old. I did have to supplement with formula at 5 months when I went back to work. It is a challenging decision not to vaccinate but when I see how healthy my daughter is I feel that could all be different if I had vaccinated her, the exact opposite of what the doctors say."

USA

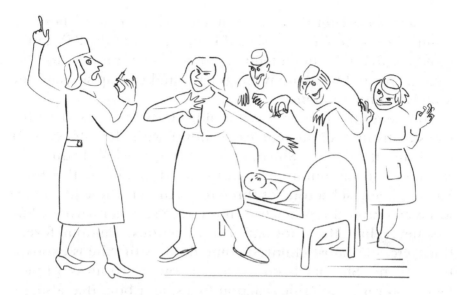

"I have had 4 children. Three of which were vaccinated with most of the vaccines. They spent their childhood with many illnesses, mostly respiratory related.

My fourth child came along later in life and after doing my own research into vaccines, as I found many changes in children's health since I was a child and the only thing I could find different was the amount of vaccines that were given. It was horrifying. When I became pregnant with my fourth child, I decided that I would not put that child through the same thing.

My daughter came early. She arrived at 30 weeks. I spent the next 6 weeks fighting with doctors and nurses at the hospital about vaccinations for her. She had no health problems, she was just small. They would not release her until I gave her the RSV vaccine. I finally let them do it so that she would be released, as they were not feeding her enough at the hospital, and she was not gaining enough weight. I attribute this to the fact that she was triple insured and she was paying for many other preemies in the NICU.

A few weeks later there was a preemie reunion at the hospital. A nurse cornered me and asked if I got the rest of the RSV series. I told her that I did not intend to, nor any other vaccines for that matter. She told me that my daughter would end up sick and she would die without them.

My daughter is now 9 years old. She was exposed to the measles from a child that came down with the illness after receiving the vaccine. She did not get the measles. By this time she was 3 so my immunity had worn off of her by this time. She has been sick a total of three times in her whole life. Once was a cold and the other two times were stomach viruses. She has never had the "normal" ear infections, random fevers, flues, etc. that most children come down with. She is exposed to everyone. She has been to the emergency room two times. Once was for an allergic reaction to a spider bite, that also got my dog who had the same reaction, and the other time for a broken arm.

She is a normal child who participates in normal activities. I can only attribute her good health with the refusal of vaccinations. Her diet is the same as my older children.

At first I used to get a hard time for my choice by many people, but that has changed. I think there are more people becoming aware of the dangers. I still have times when people want to push them, however I respond with asking them if they can list the ingredients and the side effects of those ingredients. I have had adverse reactions to two different vaccines, that I only found out well after the fact and it was too late to do anything about it. The first time I nearly died. I feel that if there is even a minuscule chance that my child will die from a chemical medication, I will not take the chance. A healthy child can fight off a disease, a child with a compromised immune system cannot, therefore it is much safer to forego the vaccines.

I also have my religious reasons for declining vaccinations, which I was not aware about prior to my research into the ingredients.

I do hope that more parents become aware of the dangers. My biggest wish is that the doctors that give these vaccines will give a list of the ingredients and ALL of the adverse reactions to parents before they administer the vaccines and allow the parents to decide whether it is worth the risk to their family."

"My wife and I have three children aged 13, 9 and 6. None are vaccinated. We have wrestled with this decision for the entire 13 years that we have been parents. We read about the lack of research on safety and effectiveness and feel confident for a time in our decision. Then we read about how childhood vaccinations have helped and we were in doubt for a while. Then we did more research and learned how vaccinations create permanent imbalances between humoral and cellular immunity and can create auto-immunity and lead to chronic diseases like asthma. Our minds are finally at ease and we are firm in our resolve.

Our three kids have not had illness-free lives. We do not exclusively eat organic food or raise our own chickens. Fast food is a part of our lives, as are school lunches. They were all breast-fed for at least a year, but did receive formula and cereal to supplement it after six months of age.

All three children get coughs, colds and flu-like illnesses in the fall and winter despite our efforts to supplement with probiotics and Vitamin D. All three had chicken pox and I suspect they all survived pertussis. But each time, I realize that this is one more virus that they will be immune to for the rest of their lives. I want them to have to fight off the bugs that go around because each time they do, they become stronger. On the other hand, the only time any of them has been to the pediatrician has been for school physicals. They don't have chronic problems, ADD or allergies. Now my oldest does have a mild form of exercise-induced asthma. He was born by C-section and my wife did have bronchitis in her 8th month of pregnancy that was treated with medication. She was also on intravenous antibiotics for three days after my son was born due to C-section complications. So I'm not surprised that my son has this issue. It is my firm belief that if we had vaccinated him, his symptoms would be much worse.

They are all bright, active and healthy. I would be devastated if by my choice to vaccinate, I had reduced their potential even a little."

"Two children, neither were vaccinated at any point during childhood. Incidence rate of sleep problems (0%), inner ear infections (0%), immune problems (0%), multiple sick days from school (very little). My daughter contracted a peanut allergy and at 18 months aspirated a seed – which led to a bronchoscopy and later asthma – but after age 10 her symptoms were minor. She still carries an inhaler, but as an adult almost never uses it. My son has never had any substantial health problems – he is now in HS. Our choice not to vaccinate, plus vitamins and organic foods from an early age, plenty of exercise, and proper health habits (posture, sleep patterns, no drug use, no alcohol) have led to very few health concerns over their lifetimes. Sports injuries – that's a different story."

"I have three extremely healthy completely unvaccinated children. I had all three of my children at home. The vaccination issue was part of our decision to give birth at home since it is so "routine" here to do these things to children without consulting the parents. We are highly educated parents. I am a medical professional and my husband is in law enforcement. My husband suffers from a major vaccine injury, which he received from the military in 2004.

I have a five-year-old son (b.10/2006), a two-year-old daughter (b.9/09) and a 1 year old son (b.3/2011). None of my children have ever had to go to the hospital or pediatrician for an illness. We don't do well-baby visits because they only want to inject them. The pediatrician told me there was no point in me coming if I was going to refuse vaccines every time so we stopped going. They've never had so much as an ear infection. No antibiotics, no medications, nothing. They've never been diagnosed with any illnesses. We get a slight cold every year that generally consists of a fever that lasts for less than 24 hours. Sometimes we'll get runny noses. Never had diarrhea or serious vomiting. They are also all-intact and have never had any surgeries.

We live in NYC and we have been denied religious waivers for vaccination so they are home schooled. It puts a lot of stress on our family to be vax free because not many people understand and families have refused to allow our children around other children. Summer camps, schools, play groups, etc. which ask for vax records have denied participation. My five-year-old tested in the gifted and talented program and is currently at a second grade level. My two-year-old is kindergarten level. They all walked early, talked early and have participated in research studies on intelligent children.

We know this is best for our children and will fight it every step of the way. When we see other children who are suffering from asthma, allergies, ear infections, surgeries to correct complications from infections, autism, disability, ADHD, ADD, behavioral issues, neurological issues, etc., we KNOW we made the best choice. I have tried to tell others to be careful about vaccines and I have warned them, particularly of the issues with ear infections, and they haven't listened. Then they call me after their children are getting tubes put in their ears asking how they can fix the damage. I always try to tell people. You can ALWAYS vax in the future once you have done more research but you can never take away damage. If my extremely healthy, intelligent children are any indication of what children COULD be without these injections, then sign me up!

Thanks for highlighting children who are not vaxed to show they aren't all injured or come from "hippy" parents who are uneducated!"

"I have 6 children. My oldest, born in 1977 received all the childhood vaccines of his day, the last ones were at 5 years old. The only good thing about this is that they were half the amount given today and he never received any as a tiny newborn or 5 at once. My second son born in 1981 received all the baby shots, but not his 5 year old or any after that. My next child was born in 1985 and received a set of shots at 10 months and that's all. My next child and first daughter was born in 1985 and at 22 years old has never had a vaccination in her life. She has never been seriously ill and I can't even remember her even having a high fever in her life. She has also never had antibiotics. She is completely normal, healthy, and beautiful and as I type this right now, she is expecting her first child with no plans to ever vaccinate her either. My next daughter was born in 1992 and at 20 years old has never been immunized. Healthy also with a daughter she doesn't intend to immunize. Never been seriously ill and I think both girls may had a light case of chicken pox. My 6th child, a son, was born in 2001 and has never been immunized either. Very healthy, never had reason for antibiotics. Healthy, healthy, healthy is all I can say."

"We have a 3-year-old son and a 1-year-old son. Neither has ever received any vaccines and they are both very healthy. The oldest has had one minor ear infection but the doctor said it wasn't bad enough to prescribe anything for, and that's it. We don't eat a perfect diet by any means, and we are not clean freaks, but yet they still seem healthier than the vaccinated children their age that we know."

USA

"Tyler was born 12/11/05. I was induced at 38 weeks due to gestational diabetes and when I opted for the epidural, the drugs made Tyler's heart rate plummet so I underwent an emergency C-section. Everything was fine after that though and we enjoy robust health with our now 6-year-old boy! We live in Eugene, Oregon USA and our culture is pretty relaxed. My husband and I were both born here and have spent the majority of our lives here, which I'm sure has contributed to our liberal views and well as a "Question Authority" frame of mind. It's all about the hippies. Anyway. When it came time for Tyler's 2 month checkup I was handed a few printouts with information regarding the barrage of vaccines my infant was about to receive. I had prepared myself to just do it. Get him vaccinated because that's just what happens. I started reading through the information and grew more hesitant. So many vaccines at such a young age? Each description also had information about the Federal Vaccine Injury Compensation Program and that really freaked me out. I thought, what the hell? There is a program that will compensate me if my infant is harmed or *killed by these vaccines*? Enough so that there is a federal compensation program? Aren't they supposed to improve the quality of our lives? No thank you. Of course that didn't go over very well with the doctor but I said that I just wasn't ready to vaccinate him and that I needed to do more research.

After that my resolve just grew. It seemed that there was one side which was very big government and big company and that it was a formatted response. Then there was the side that was really questioning and even downright saying it's dangerous, don't do it. Dr. Mercola and Jane Burgermeister have presented lots of information which is contrary to what the CDC, AMA, and AAP all vehemently agree upon even though there has been almost no research to prove the efficacy and safety of vaccines. I've also been very interested in the vaccine-autism connection and was especially gratified by watching Dr. Mercola's interview with Dr. Wakefield.

Tyler has energy that rarely wanes, is extraordinarily creative and heart touchingly kind. He has been sick a few times usually a stomach or flu bug which he usually is over in a day or 2. One thing I've done to help him stay healthy is to use lavender and peppermint essential oils, too. They seem to help out a lot, smell great and are chemical free. He is tall for his age, solidly built and enjoys natural grace and balance. He loves to sing and dance and is always ready for a joke and a laugh, he is truly a joy!

We are very lucky to live in a community with one of the cleanest water supplies in the world. We are also fortunate that organic food is a big deal here and Tyler is being raised with some of the best quality food and water on earth which surely contributes to his excellent health."

"Here's my story about unvaccinated children. I'm 27 years old. Come from a family of 6 where all kids were not vaccinated. My parents raised us on very healthy foods. Whole grains, beans, lot's of vegetables and good quality soy sauce, miso, sea weeds. We were always in great health. As a child I had minor cases of 5 of the common child diseases. Measles, chicken pox, whooping cough, German measles (rubella), mumps. As I said they where all very mild cases and I had no further complications.

As of now I'm still in great health. I'm raising my 4 kids this natural way. They are very healthy. Two years ago they had a mild case of chicken pox. Also my sister who just had her 3rd baby is not vaccinating. And my dad came from a family of 5 where no one was vaccinated either. You may say... It runs in the family."

USA

"I have two unvaccinated girls, ages 4 and 6. I have nothing much to report, they have no health issues, maybe a couple mild ear aches, they both have thrown up/had diarrhea only a couple times while sick (except for the time we did get rotavirus). Other than that, they are totally healthy. I do find it odd that my friend's children seem to have all sorts of issues, such as allergies, having their tonsils removed, nebulizers, learning or cognitive disabilities, etc. And it is accepted as perfectly normal? The sad truth it has become the norm.

We looked into vaccines after my stepson, age 9 now, started regressing at 18 months and developed, what was later diagnosed, autism."

"My son is a happy, healthy and vibrant 4-year old. He was born at home, eats mainly organic and natural foods, never was vaccinated and will most likely be home-schooled. My husband and I did not come to the decision to not vaccinate lightly. We spent countless hours researching, watching lectures, reading stories and watching documentaries. Actually, the more we learned the more we became angry and frustrated so many others do not question the medical and pharmaceutical industries. They are literally destroying our children, and we need to continue to bring awareness to this issue. It deeply saddens me that many are so unwilling to question science and better understand how immunity actually works. Thank goodness I listened to my maternal intuition; my son can thank me for it. He is rarely ever sick, and if he is it is usual very mild and over in a few days. He has never been to the doctor for an illness, we take him to the chiropractor instead. He is thriving and beautiful."

"I have 9 children. Four of them are fully vaccinated, two are partially vaccinated, and 3 are not vaccinated at all. 8 of my 9 children (including the vaccinated ones) contracted chicken pox, and it was mild in all of them. One of my unvaccinated children contracted measles, and it was even milder than the chicken pox. It makes me wonder what all the hullabaloo is about, probably because the disease takes about 10 days to run its course, and no one wants to miss that much work or school. Interestingly, my other 2 unvaccinated kids didn't catch the measles from him. Two of my kids contracted pertussis (whooping cough), one vaccinated and one unvaccinated. Interestingly, the unvaccinated daughter kicked it more easily than the vaccinated son, who struggled even a year later with coughing spells!

Some may question my sanity, knowing my kids contracted whooping cough yet still sticking to the decision to not vaccinate. Well, my daughter is alive and healthy. Unfortunately my sister's nephew (on her husband's side) died in his car seat on the way home from having a DPT shot. When his mommy went to get him out of his car seat when they arrived home, her baby was dead, and all her efforts to resuscitate him were to no avail (she was a nurse). Because of this extreme reaction, my sister's children aren't allowed to have the pertussis vaccine. But, that's not a problem, since the disease is fairly easy to treat. My kids, other than the rare cold and even rarer flu, are never sick - except for the instances I mentioned (which has been spread over 28 years). I will be honest with you - we aren't on the healthiest diet. My kids enjoy junk food and McDonald's food and Lucky Charms for breakfast - and they're STILL healthier than all their friends!"

"I am mom to five children, ages 22, 19, 16, 13, and 8. None are vaccinated, and the only children I know who are as healthy as they are belong to other families who also decided not to vaccinate. Only the three youngest are now living at home, but of those three, NONE have ever needed to go to a doctor. Not once. They have gone for a couple of physicals that were needed to play sports, and always got a clean bill of health. They were born at home. I also breastfed them for 2.5-4.5 years, so that probably aided their health too. It makes me sad to see how much time most of my friends' kids spend at the doctor. I am so happy that I had time to research it before I had my first child. That first child did end up having a slew of vaccinations when he joined the Air Force (which made him very sick for short time), but at least he had an adult body weight to deal with all that gunk."

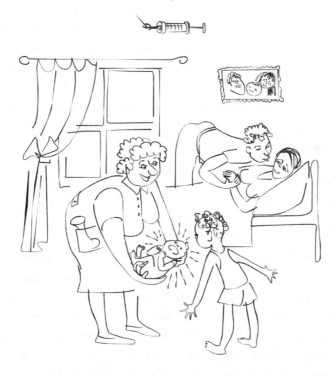

"My two boys are totally unvaccinated and very healthy. Our oldest was born in a hospital when we really did not have the courage to have him at home. With our birth plan well known, the doctors never pushed us to vaccinate, but they did want to give him a vitamin K shot. We said no. Our youngest was born at home, in his own bedroom, with a midwife. No drugs, just a natural delivery, as it was with our first. They are both wonderful, smart, active and healthy children. They go to a public school and despite what people seem to think sometimes, they do not need vaccinations to go to school.

The only time a needle has been near either one of them was when my oldest decided to lie down on his skateboard heading downhill and got too close to a parked car. He split his upper arm open and needed stitches. They numbed the area before cleaning it and stitching him back up. His mother and I decided long ago, if they ever mandated vaccinations for them, we would rather move than give them to them. Thank God for our freedoms and our choices we have with the exemptions. Having both parents as doctors definitely helps our kids out as we are knowledgeable as how to help our children succeed and be healthy. Eating right, exercise, getting good rest and regular chiropractic care are all very important to our kids' healthy lives."

Jason Williamson DC, Great Lakes Family Chiropractic, www.drjasonw.com

"My 3 year old daughter has not received any vaccinations. She is healthy and smart and has attended daycare since she was 18 months old. She only drinks raw milk and has never taken Tylenol or antibiotics. She has no asthma, allergies, or eczema. She recovers from colds quickly. She had bronchitis once, but was better within 3 days and it did not reoccur. She's gotten a few ear infections that were cured with garlic oil. Overall she is in super health and I am very happy with my decision not to have her vaccinated!"

"I am a mother of 4 girls......8, 6, 4 and 1. I was very educated from day one of conceiving my first child. I graduated with a degree in Human Biology and a Doctorate in Chiropractic. I knew from the beginning that I was NOT vaccinating my children or giving them any drugs unless absolutely necessary. To date, none of my girls have received a vaccine, they have never been prescribed an antibiotic for infection, nor have I given them any fever reducing drugs. All 4 girls are very healthy, never missing school or school functions. We do not make trips to the pediatrician......for anything! They do come down with a common cold every once in awhile or a very rare case of the puke germ; otherwise, these girls just do not get sick! I contribute their health partly to not being vaccinated. Being a Chiropractor, I do adjust their spines and feed them very well with the right foods, which also contributes to their health.

Currently, I have two girls going to public school and they excel scholastically receiving all A's. All 4 girls were verbal at an early age, speaking clear and forming sentences. They seem to do very well with fine and gross motor skills as well.

I see so many children through my occupation that have been fully vaccinated; usually have food sensitivities, and/or seasonal allergies. I have worked with a Medical Doctor that treats autism and saw in many situations a direct relation to vaccinations and bad reactions. Seeing these patients on a regular basis confirms my decision of not vaccinating."

Kelly L. Borchers, D.C., Valley Health Center, D.C. 423 West Main St., Tipp City, OH 45371, 937.667.2222

"We are writing this story to let others see how making the choice to not vaccinate our daughter was the best choice for us. My daughter was born Feb 15 2009 at 6 lbs 10 oz healthy and full term. I breastfed her only. She was a great baby sleeping through the night at 3 weeks old! She continued to be a healthy, happy baby at 4 months she holds sippy cup and drinks water. By 6 months she is saying and using sign language mama milk dada and by 9 months she was walking. She is now 3 years old and we can say that she has only had a cold once since she has been born. She weighs 29 pounds and is 37 inches tall. She talks in full sentences and is striving and thriving in all that she does. We as her parents can say without a shadow of a doubt that we made the best choice not to vaccinate her. We did our homework while pregnant and read many books and talked to many different doctors about our choice and we continue to educate ourselves and others around us to think about their choices as a parent and make an informed decision on what is best for you and your family!"

"Haven, our three year old daughter, has never been vaccinated and is in outstanding health. She has only been to the doctor twice; once for a normal wellness check-up and once for teething pain. She has been in daycare since she was 6 months old and has rarely been sick. One time she caught the flu, signs of which began to show one evening as she complained of a tummy ache. She vomited twice that night and then awoke in the morning ready to eat and play. She's had 2-3 colds, but they have never gotten any worse than a little clear runny nose and cough. They lasted around 3 days each. Her daycare had an outbreak of Hand, Foot, and Mouth disease as well as a couple of children with Rotavirus. She never caught any of them. Her immunity has been very strong, thank God. We give her acidophilus daily and frequently kefir, as well as eating organic. She's never had fast food, sodas, or candy. She only gets cupcakes at birthday parties and has only had juice once or twice. We also don't watch TV and try to stay as active as possible, engaging her in daily walks or swimming. We've been very blessed to see her grow up as an active, healthy three year old who has also been very advanced in her learning. We certainly don't regret not having vaccinated her, especially since most of the diseases they're vaccinated for are ones they are only susceptible to before the age of 2."

"I was blessed that shortly after my first son was born, another couple with a newborn asked me if we were going to vaccinate him. Until then, I had never heard of people not vaccinating their children. We just assumed that it was good and that it is what everyone should do. I started studying about vaccines. By my son's first checkup, I was sure we did not want to vaccinate. The doctors gave me such a horrible time in their office, that after two hours of interrogation and tears, my husband and I gave in and we allowed three vaccines that day. That experience was awful and we almost decided just to vaccinate like the majority.

However, as God would have it, I was invited to a class on homeopathy at our local food co-op the day before my first son was supposed to receive his second round of shots. During the class, the homeopath started talking about vaccines and everything he taught us made sense. I went home and spent the rest of that day researching vaccination. When my husband came home from work, the entire upstairs was covered in documents. We decided that evening – no shots. I have been studying vaccines ever since. This quest to understand vaccines led me to a career in homeopathy. After my receiving my BA degree, I returned to school and graduated from the Northwestern Academy of Homeopathy - a four-year homeopathic academy in Minnesota.

That single question that those parents asked us about whether we would vaccinate our baby has really taken our family on a journey. It has taken me twelve years to come to a knowing in my soul about exactly what it is that I believe about vaccines. I can understand why people used to believe in vaccines and why it seemed to be a good idea. I am now content to reason that vaccines might be good in some cases. I am not in a camp that believes they are all bad. I do know that we have been fed many untruths about the successes of vaccination and that the diseases that vaccines have been given credit for eradicating have actually taken care of themselves before vaccines for them were ever developed. I have decided that even though there may be some benefit to a vaccine, in the big picture the DNA, viruses/diseases and toxins that we are putting into our bloodstream, are more dangerous and devastating for our long-term health that the possible benefits that any vaccine may offer. For me, it is now a matter of deciding not whether vaccines are "good or bad" but it is about deciding what is the least harmful option for my children. This understanding about our choice to not vaccinate has given me the most peace. This is something that most parents can understand. Parents are supposed to protect their children. We do our best.

I have four children who are all not vaccinated. They are 13, 10, 8 and 6 years old now. With the exception of my son who feels like he needs to keep breaking his arms and one ear infection when my daughter was 4 years old, none of them has ever had any reason to go to a doctor. We do not have any eczema, psoriasis, asthma, or allergies. They are not autistic and they do not have any learning disorders.

My sister has three children. Two of them so far who are both fully-vaccinated have asthma. Her second born not only has asthma, but also food allergies and intense skin-rash issues. I do not know what they have done for their third child, but I was told they are considering stopping all of their vaccines. Our neighbor has an autistic daughter who was a normal sweet little girl that could talk and play like any other child until her MMR vaccine. One month later she stopped talking and interacting. Very sad.

I am thankful every day that we did not vaccinate. My children are happy and healthy. Needless to say they are very educated about vaccines and are passionate about this topic. I still do not take my children's health for granted. We also try to do as much organic food as possible and we have a farmer who supplies us with organic raw milk, cheese and meats. I have always dreamed that someone would do a study on the health of unvaccinated children.

I am so thankful that you are compiling information for the world to see. We can only hope that our family is a good example of how healthy children can be without the toxins in their system. We have been blessed!"

"I was 19 years old when my son was born and two years later I gave birth to my first daughter. Both of these children were vaccinated like clockwork. Both of my older children developed all the "normal" childhood illnesses and some not so normal childhood illnesses. My son got the usual suspects: lots of ear infections, sick all the time, fevers. The doctor was constantly putting him on antibiotics and we almost got tubes put into his ears. He was later diagnosed with dyslexia.

My daughter was frequently sick also. At one point, my daughter was so sick, the doctor did not know what was wrong with her and we ended up in the hospital for a spinal tap. I think she was about 4 or 5 months old, and no, she did not have spinal meningitis.

Never did any doctor inform me there might be side effects to vaccinations.

Along came child number 3, which was about the time that I stopped vaccinating my children in 1983, so my son was four, one daughter was two and my youngest was just a newborn. The newborn got one or two vaccinations and then that was it. No more vaccinations.

In 1988, I had my fourth child and she was born at home and never vaccinated. My two youngest daughters never got the "normal" childhood illnesses. My third child just never got sick; the youngest had a stomach ailment once where she threw up everything and anything except breast milk. At the time she was about 2 years old. I nursed her regularly and would attempt to feed her one food at a time (without success). She was sick like this for about 3 weeks and then it went away and everything was fine. The baby also got a case of impetigo, which did call for the use of antibiotics.

The differences between the two older children and the two youngest children were remarkable in that the older kids were always sick and the two younger children were so rarely sick.

I have also seen the same results with my grandchildren. My son's first two children were fully vaccinated for the first 4 or 5 years and they were always sick with oldest child having learning disabilities. The third child was not vaccinated, and she was sick a lot less than her brothers. Once my daughter-in-law took the kids off dairy and wheat we saw a huge difference in their behavior and in their health!

My daughters did not vaccinate their children and guess what? No chronic ear infections, no chronic upper respiratory illnesses, no learning disabilities - so far!

My fiancé's daughter recently vaccinated her son and guess what? The child had a seizure two weeks later and the doctor told her that was "normal."

Yes, I suppose chronically sick kids having seizures and learning disabilities is the new "normal." What a pity. MD's don't really know what a healthy child looks like anymore!"

"I have a four year old daughter who is not vaccinated...only had the vitamin K shot, which they did without asking. She was raised on formula and her diet is not the best. (My wife and I do not see eye to eye on this issue, among others...diet being another big one (too much sugar and not enough raw food. It's a compromise. If that's what it takes to stave off the shots then so be it.) She has agreed to not getting her vaccinated ONLY because she has a relative that had a child that died after an MMR shot. Anyway....My daughter has had many visits to the doctor for ear infections and strep. Antibiotics were administered. The first three years were the worst but the trips to the doc are getting fewer and further between. The last trip, the doc said she may have asthma. I don't buy it. She was given a prescription and took it a few times but we have pretty much weaned her off of it. We have a cat that she may be allergic to so it has been banished to the outdoors. Daughter seems fine now. Mentally she is a wonderful child, very smart and talkative, loving and learns fast. She seems more developed than a lot of children her age.

I believe she would have never had gotten sick if she had been breast fed, ate right etc. I am 40. I had some shots but not many. I haven't had a shot in 30 years and I very seldom get sick. I got sick some when I was younger but nothing out of the ordinary. I was also bottle-fed. Eventually your immune system will catch up if you were bottle-fed, it just takes longer.

Nowadays, the combination of shots, bad diet, and formula fed is a recipe for disaster."

"As a mother of an unvaccinated child, I am grateful and relieved that I investigated and researched childhood vaccinations before I gave birth to my child. I was able to make an informed choice to keep my son vaccine free when the hospital suggested the Hepatitis B shot at birth. I was also able to know that I, myself, should decline the rubella booster they tried to give me in the hospital when my son was born as well. The rubella vaccine could have transferred to my son through breast milk and potentially caused adverse effects on his immune system.

My son hasn't been sick in almost six months even though he has been exposed to colds from his babysitter. It seems as if his immune system is naturally maturing in a positive manner. When he was a baby he did get the flu twice, but both bouts of the sickness lasted only a day. He was running around, with energy mind you, while the others who had it were bed-ridden. He also caught roseola at about 16 months old, which was the most sick he has ever been. I took him to the doctor and they didn't even diagnose him with it. It was apparent he had it after his sickness had passed and the rash appeared and then disappeared for a day. Even though he caught that childhood disease I never wavered in my conviction that his body could handle childhood diseases. As long as a parent cares for their child and keeps their temperatures down, and keeps fluid in them, they will most likely make it through.

My son has never had one ear infection; he has never been on antibiotics for anything. When he has been sick in the past, except for the roseola episode, he was literally running around with his boundless energy and the only way you can tell he was sick was because he vomited. He is alert, says hundreds of words, is bright-eyed, very social, very active and pretty much has always been ahead of all his milestones. In fact, when we go out in public, he seems much more alert and social than many of the other kids. He will go up to kids on the playground and try to initiate play with them, while most of the kids seem adverse to interaction from him. He has never had a drippy, running nose like many children I have seen. I have talked to some parents of vaccinated children who have informed me that their children's noses seem to drip incessantly, never stopping, even though they appear healthy.

My brother has seven children, his last three of whom are not vaccinated. One of his daughters, who is in kindergarten, rarely gets sick, while her vaccinated brothers and sisters do more often. She remains healthy while they have colds and flus. She has caught strep throat, but was treated with antibiotics, and did fine. When she caught strep throat after first attending kindergarten that was the first time she had been sick in years.

At first my family didn't understand why I chose to not vaccinate my son, but now they all back me 100 percent. My son's father has always supported the non-vaccination route. We have a relatively understanding health care insurance plan with Kaiser and they don't harass me on my choice. I switched doctors in the beginning because my son's first pediatrician seemed put off by my choice. Now his doctor is completely understanding of our choice and doesn't even question me. I also don't take him in for well visits because it is apparent to everyone that my son is very healthy, and I don't feel the need to have to deny the shots the visits are intended for."

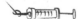

"My unvaccinated daughter just turned 9 years old. All I can say is her health is incredible despite the fact that I had to stop breast-feeding her after 2 weeks of age. My 3 other vaccinated children whom I nursed between 9 and 22 months were never as healthy especially in the first 5 years of life. My daughter has zero learning disabilities. She is athletic. She loves music and art and has friends galore.

I try very hard to feed my children a healthy diet and I make everything from scratch. We drink raw milk and bone broths. I sprout, grind and soak my grains. However, my unvaccinated daughter loves junk food and at parties she doesn't hold back. Yet she doesn't get sick. I treat all my children using homeopathic medicine, herbs and rest when they have colds or infections. We do not use any pharmaceutical products."

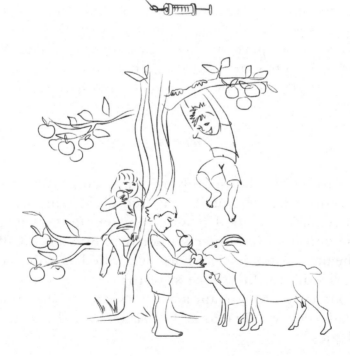

"Actually our story is very simple and basic. Our three completely natural, vaccine-free grandchildren, Thomas 7, William 5, and

Naomi 3, were born via natural childbirth, nursed until they weaned themselves at ages 2, 2, and 1 respectively, and are raised on organic vegetables and fruits, as well as organic home grown meats, whole grains, raw honey, plenty of berries, nuts, and seeds. Two of the kids love raw goat milk and goat cheese.

William used to react to cow and goat milk products, peanut butter, and certain types of fish. He reacted by vomiting within a few minutes after eating any of those foods. According to the last allergy test, he now reacts only to fish. William also has a mild type of asthma for which he does use medicine when needed.

Overall I would consider all three of my grandchildren very healthy. When they have a cold they get over it in a day or two. As far as childhood diseases, they have been exposed to chicken pox several times but must have immunity since they never had any of the symptoms."

Their teeth are perfect. No cavities in any of them. We have no fluoride in our water and use natural toothpaste. None of the kids wear glasses. They are just cheerful, happy, bright kids. That's it!"

"I have one child almost fully vaxed & cured of an autism spectrum disorder. My totally unvaxed child (she just turned 16) has remarkably good health. She has never had an ear infection and not even one cold per year. She has no allergies or any health-related issues whatsoever. She has only been to a doctor twice in her life (once at birth) because she has never been sick enough to warrant a doctor's visit. I know for a fact if she had been vaccinated as her sister was, she would have health issues."

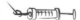

"I have 3 beautiful, healthy, children, ages 10, 8, and 2. Being born in California, they all were required to receive a "vitamin K" shot, I was told by the nurse there. They've never had any other vaccinations and are all very healthy, with the exception of the snotty nose on occasion. Anywhere I've been with the kids, I usually get comments on how "well adjusted" they are.

I do buy all organic natural foods, grass fed beef, range chicken, raw cow milk, and distilled water is used in all food prep and beverages, which I believe makes a big difference in overall health. I don't look at the cost of foods but I pay zero medical expenses other than dental care."

"I am chiropractor. Many people think that means I am simply anti-anything medical. That is not the case. I felt with the knowledge I had and the information I had seen before I had kids, it was my responsibility to do my own homework and then decide on my own.

After review of the information, I truly felt that vaccines were given too much credit for eliminating and / or curing diseases. I also determined that injecting the many toxins directly into the bloodstream could pose a risk.

I did not vaccinate any of my 3 kids. As of March 2012, my 3 kids are 10, 8, and 4. Three boys that have NEVER been vaccinated. They also have never had an ear infection. Now, with me being a chiropractic dad, I adjust my kids for health and wellness. This does not mean they have an invisible shield, but in comparison to our friends with kids the same age, my kids are just about never sick.

When my kids get a cold - this has happened about once every 2-3 years - the cold and or fever lasts for about 1/2 day and then it passes and is done. My kids almost never miss school. As far as vaccine related "diseases", they did all get the chicken pox. Again, very mild and my kids never felt sick, had a fever and lasted a short period of time.

My three children are excelling in school and all are in better overall health then their friends. Funny, there is a family across the street and we carpool. All 6 kids together, in the same car, go to the same school and they are frequently at our house and vice versa. Now those kids have missed a lot of school this year. One kid has missed 15 times and is frequently sick. Their grandfather is a PA (physician's assistant) and made sure to protect the family with FLU shots. 2-3 weeks after the flu shots, 2 of 3 kids got the flu.

My kids are very active, love school and have a very upbeat attitude. They look forward to life. As a chiropractor, I have seen many kids that were fine, then they were vaccinated and they "changed". It is very sad to see an autistic kid or a neurologically damaged child. Most parents that I interact with are big on the flu shots, antibiotics and meds immediately when there is a sniffle.

I can't say enough on how awesome the health of my kids is. I am glad that I did not subscribe to - in my opinion - propaganda and junk science regarding vaccines. I will say that my oldest will be 11 this year. He would have had a play-buddy that was a friend of mine, but the boy was vaccinated and after a series of vaccines, died.

He blamed the vaccines and the doctor said that he (the father) must have done something and was going to report him to the police. His son died from a reaction to a vaccine.

I will never allow my children to be poisoned. I challenge all the CEO's of the vaccines to get an equivalent dose if they are so safe."

"I'm not 100% sure why my mom isn't vaccinated but I think it has to do with my uncle, her older brother, falling out of a moving car. He had a head injury and couldn't function like he had previously. My grandparents went to every medical specialist to figure out how to make him better. Someone told them about a chiropractor and as a last resort they carried my uncle into her office and he was able to walk out! After that my grandpa went to Palmer chiropractic school. I think he figured if a chiropractor could fix his son when no medical doctor could then chiropractic care could fix anything.

My mom's reasoning is a little different and has to do with her younger brothers. She is number 5 of 7 kids. She's still chiropractic, we all are, but when my grandma went into labor they gave her twilight sleep, or something, it was supposed to help with the pain and it stopped her labor putting the baby into distress but they didn't know that till after he was born. He almost died and had cerebral palsy as a result. We have babies without pain meds now. My mom's fear of that situation repeating is pretty ingrained in all of us. So my mom talks about that being a reason but also because we're a chiropractic family. My kids have been healthier than a lot of kids we know and the people who know we don't vaccinate call me every time there is a whisper of an outbreak, so we just assure them we're fine and go to the chiropractor more then usual. My reasons are my mom and my grandma. My siblings and I have never had major illnesses, no surgeries, no tubes in our ears and that is testimony enough for me to keep my kids safe from all the junk they want to inject into my few-hour-old innocent babies."

"The delivery was a story itself. The ending is the best part. Steele literally shot out of mom and the midwife had to catch her in mid air. The look on her face was priceless. Being a Maximized Living Doctor I immediately checked her spine for any problems, which there was so I adjusted it. She was nursing and sleeping on and off for hours. We were all in our bed at home, at peace and in awe of what God had done.

There was absolutely no human intervention during the entire process. There were no ultrasounds, no fasting glucose tests, nothing. Steele is 9 months now, has breast fed the entire time, has been eating solid organic food for over a month and was walking or trying to at 8.5 months. She now runs. Her favorite thing to do apart from chasing mom and dad around is to read by herself. She will sit there in the middle of the living room with a book and shout like she is reading.

Both myself and mom were not very healthy as children. I was sick when I was born and stayed that way until 13 constantly at the doctor's office for horrific asthma and allergies. We were both vaccinated. I did not have my spine corrected until 13 and mom until she was 30 (before pregnancy). Today, we both have incredible health.

This baby however has health from another stratosphere. Her skin is flawless. Her poops are smooth and all the time. She slept through the night immediately. Now she wakes up to eat sometimes but only then. She has had a runny nose during teething and while her body is figuring things out. And we do not even have a thermometer. There is no pediatrician. She is growing up without thinking she has to go to a doctor for any other reason than an emergency. How cool is that!!!

She is around other kids all the time. One time we had a real sick little baby make an emergency visit to our house for an adjustment. She was feverish, snot coming from everywhere and not happy. The parents were a little worried about having her around our baby. We were not. In fact, we knew that if Steele did get feverish after being around this ill child that it would be good for her body! She never even got a snotty nose.

Her best friend and cousin both were born a few months before. Both of them found out we were not vaccinating and they decided not to either! Both of them had their spine checked at birth. We now have these three girls running around incredibly healthy and not sick! Steele has cut herself and not gotten infected. Her cousin pulled a curling iron onto her arm, did not get infected, healed up just fine with no scarring. There have been no ear infections, no crying all night because of pain.

As I am writing this I just thought of taking my sweet girl to a doctor and having them come at her with a needle. She would look at me as if to say, "WHY DADDY!" I cannot explain the rage that would come over me if a doctor even suggested that to us.

Steele, her cousin and best friend are living proof that vaccines are not necessary. I have family who labeled us crazy...until they saw this beautiful baby. The shock that she is healthy has brought them to the light.

I hope this letter helps someone because vaccines are unholy, they are an assault on a human and the profiteers from them will answer for their crimes in this life or the next."

"After doing an enormous amount of research on vaccines and talking with our pediatrician, we decided to focus on keeping our son's immune system strong rather than vaccinating and we are seeing the rewards. Our son is now 9 and he has always been extremely healthy, no ear infections, no asthma, no allergies, just an occasional cold. He always recovers within a couple of days. When we asked our pediatrician about the whooping cough (pertussis) that was going around, he told us that all of the kids he has seen who had it were vaccinated for it. The kids who were not vaccinated for it were not catching it! We are hoping to be able to expose him to chicken pox at an early age when it is much milder and he will get a life long, natural immunity to it like I got when I was a child and my mom took me to a chicken pox party."

"A little over ten years ago, my niece received one of her scheduled vaccination shots at her one-year checkup. Up to that point, my sister had fully followed the recommended vaccination schedule. Within twenty-four hours of receiving the shot my niece had a fever of 106 and was having febrile seizures. A violent bumpy rash appeared all over her body. She had the fever for several days. The doctor told my sister that it was impossible that it was a vaccine reaction and that she must have AIDS or leukemia. So my sister had to have her baby tested and wait for the results. Not surprisingly, they came back negative. At that point, she became very concerned and decided to do research on her own about vaccinations, and she shared the information she found with the family. Though the older grandkids were vaccinated, after that happened to my niece everyone in our family took a long, hard look at whether they were willing to risk their children. In our family now, only the kids older than my niece are fully or partially vaccinated. Any born after that happened to my niece are vaccination-free. None of the kids have died of chicken pox, whooping cough, or measles. All have good health and are very intelligent for their various ages. My niece has chronic eczema and an anxiety disorder as well as being considered pre-diabetic.

I did not allow this family experience to decide whether I was willing to vaccinate. I enjoy reading and researching just about any subject so I proceeded to do that with vaccinations. It was not an easy decision to make, or one I made lightly. I still worry and rethink and consider every angle over and over to be sure it's the right one, but we have chosen not to vaccinate our child. I have been treated by medical professionals as though I am an ignorant and careless parent because of this decision. I have been bullied, I have been lied to, and I have been threatened by doctors. I have been given deliberate misinformation in attempts to frighten me into giving my son a shot that I feel poses more of a danger to him than the disease it's supposed to protect him against.

I'm not going to go into a detailed recounting of experience after experience. Keeping it brief, my son is now just past two. He has had perhaps six or seven colds in his entire life. On average they last perhaps five days. He has had a cough, once, that lasted for a week after the other cold symptoms disappeared. After he turned two, he had his very first fever, a whopping 100.9 that lasted less than 12 hours. When he's sick, he tends to eat much more fruit and toast and avoid any eggs or meat on his plate, but he always plays and is still bright-eyed and talkative. He had thrush once after an antibiotic they gave him after birth, and he had problems with constipation for a couple months after I started him on solid foods. Aside from the colds those are the only problems with his health my son has ever had.

That being said, I have been very very careful of his diet and nutrition. He was solely breastfed until I started him on solid foods at 6 months and introduced one new food a week till he was just over one year. He still breastfeeds at night. He has never tasted formula. I waited till he was one to give him egg white, wheat, and dairy, and till he was two to allow him to have peanut butter and honey (two of his cousins have a peanut allergy so I wanted to be careful). He has never had a food allergy, but a couple of foods (cinnamon, jalapeno, spicy sausage) have given him a light contact rash on his skin that disappears within 10 minutes of cleaning his face. You may think it's odd that I allow my two year old to have foods like that but he likes everything. He eats sautéed mushrooms and onions by the handful. I have been very careful also of his sugar and dairy intake. He drinks water, or occasionally I will make him unsweetened chamomile tea or let him have almond milk. He eats lots of vegetables and whole grains, he's had McDonalds maybe twice in his life, and he only has dessert as a treat on special occasions. I let him eat all the fruit he wants, but I limit his dairy because the pediatrician said there is a connection between children with high dairy intake and severe ear infections. My son has never had an ear infection. I give him a daily kids' vitamin and whenever he's been around someone sick I give him a little extra Vitamin C and D.

As far as his mental development goes, he was bright and alert from birth. His current speech and vocabulary is closer to a three-year-old's though he just recently turned two. He is stringing together four and five word sentences, he can count to eleven, and he can recite the alphabet A-F (and he also knows H-P but for some reason skips the G). He chats on the phone with his cousins and when I give him simple three-step verbal instructions for a new activity without demonstrating visually (dip the brush in the water, then in the paint, and then put it on the paper) he comprehends and does it without prompting. He is active, friendly, social, and already has a sense of humor. I truly and sincerely believe that if we had chosen to follow the recommended vaccination schedule he would be a different child."

"I was wary of vaccines because I had a reaction to the TB test as a child & I distinctly remember being vaccinated the first time & cried & screamed the next time they tried to do it. I was also sick a lot as a child and almost died from pneumonia at age 2. When my son was born almost 5 years ago, I spent months researching everything I could regarding vaccines, what I found angered & saddened me. I read way too many horror stories of adverse vaccine reactions in perfectly healthy children. I quickly realized that the vaccines scared me way more than the diseases that they supposedly prevent. I decided that he would never receive a vaccine if I could possibly help it.

I am very happy to report that my son is one of the healthiest children I know. He has gotten a cold almost every year of his life but he is usually over it in a couple of days and you really wouldn't even know he was sick except for a runny nose & fever because he doesn't act like he even feels bad. We only visit the doctor for well checks. He is very advanced for his age, sweet and happy and truly a joy to be around. I can't say for sure that things would be different if he had been vaccinated but I truly believe that my decision to breastfeed, not circumcise, feed him healthy organic foods & not vaccinate him at all have contributed to the healthy, happy child he is today.

Thank you so much for doing this survey that for some reason [???] the pharmaceutical companies refuse to do. I am happy to participate in anything else that may help enlighten people to the truth. It breaks my heart on a daily basis that children are subjected to these poisons that can kill or maim them for life. I am thankful that I listened to my intuition and did my homework on this subject."

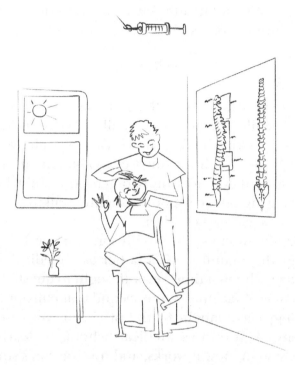

"My daughter was born in a hospital even though I would have preferred a water birth. She did not receive any of the birth vaccines, no vitamin k shot and I declined all the tests they like to do a few days after birth, such as hearing, etc. We feel strongly that when a baby is born, they need peace and quiet to help them and their bodies settle in to their new body and environment. My daughter is now 6 years old and has lived an organic, natural lifestyle. She has never had any vaccines, medications, over the counter drugs and no McDonalds! She is home schooled and has traveled all over the world easily. She does not have any symptoms or chronic diseases. She does not go to the medical doctor at all. We visit a Chiropractic Doctor to get adjusted periodically. My daughter is very happy and has a lot of outside time in nature and being free to explore. She knows some Spanish and we are a close knit family. She visits her grandparents on the weekends, which she looks forward to a lot. We hope that our conscious effort to provide a successful and healthy environment will pay off with our daughter's future happiness."

"It is refreshing to be asked "So, how has the decision to not vaccinate your child affected your family?" Why is it, that no one has ever asked us that before now? We have always been met with deer-in-the-head-light or quiet eyes-of-judgment, that we are making a decision that is not only wrong for our child, but risky for society by us having our "cesspool" daughter walking among them and their fully vaccinated children.

I am a family wellness-based chiropractor for 19 years. I was raised in a medical family with a father as a medical doctor and mother a nurse. The first time I ever thought to question the safety and effectiveness of vaccines was in second year chiropractic school in Immunology class, taught by the professor who also taught at the University of Toronto's Medical School. In learning about the immune system, how it works, and how vaccines stimulate the various pathways within it, vaccinations started to seem like a bad idea to me. That was 22 years ago. A lot more is known about the psychoneuroimmune system now that just reaffirms my initial questioning. I am fortunate that I knew what my decision would be regarding vaccination and raising children well before I ever had my own. Thankfully, I found a husband who completely agrees.

Our daughter is now an amazing, happy, healthy girl, never had a drug of any kind in her 10-year old life. She is healthier than I ever imagined she would be.

All of our lifestyle choices have resulted in this, not just not vaccinating. She did have a traumatic birth, was adjusted immediately and has been her whole life; breastfed for 4.5 years; we eat the best we can most of the time; she has had fevers, especially when younger, which we supported and let do their job.

She did see a medical doctor at the age of 2, foolish choice on our part, but we thought that if there was ever an emergency, we would need one. She berated us about not vaccinating, and told us our daughter was underweight, we should feed her ice cream and then come back in 2 months and they'd re-weigh her. Of course we've never been back.

All that said, I have found that the majority of parents in my practice who have made the choice to not vaccinate are well-educated and keep themselves well-informed regarding all the other health choices that are the huge responsibility of becoming a parent. It's not an easy task!"

"In 1979, before the birth of my first daughter, I had the opportunity to research vaccines and also learn about the benefits of "natural immunity". My husband, Sam, was a chiropractic student attending Sherman College of Chiropractic. We also had the privilege of meeting Dr. Robert Mendelsohn, renowned pediatrician, who wrote The Medical Heretic and several books exposing the problems with the allopathic medical model of "sickness care". That began my personal passionate journey I am still on today that I refer to as the "Vaccine Education Revolution".

I have five very healthy un-vaccinated children who are now grown young adults and starting their own families. From 1980 forward, my goal was to raise my children as natural and as healthy as I believe God intended! I birthed 4 of them at home with midwives, utilized chiropractic to tune-up their bodies when needed, and from birth forward, they were normal, bright, nurtured and protected from anything that would cause them harm within reason. I loved my children like most parents do, wanting the very best for them and also trying to avoid any of the pit-falls I went through.

We all want our children to be healthy because we all realize that health is the one gift that allows us to do virtually anything we want to do in life! Without our health, we must struggle to do even the simple things. Children, for sure, deserve the best opportunity to be healthy! We were very blessed because before our first child was born, we discovered the real secrets to raising healthy happy children!

It is not so much "what you do" but more about "what you don't do". We did things very non- traditionally....more like they would have done 100 years ago! Our children were easy to learn, happy and emotionally stable, rational and pretty easy to control with discipline. They were normal children all with unique personalities. My husband, Sam and I were on the same page with how we were going to feed them, educate them and basically, we did things a little different than most. We believe in long-term breastfeeding, the family bed, home education and avoided all medications, even over-the-counter drugs. We gave the body time to work through problems because we understood this process called immune system development. We never had a chronically sick child who needed lots of medical care. We also did not employ a pediatrician or have a plastic card referred to as "health insurance" which I believe is really the road to sickness assurance.

Sure our children got the "normal childhood illnesses" like chicken pox, runny noses and colds, swollen glands, fevers and rashes and they got sick like most. In fact, my second child, Austin, was very sensitive and was the one who had some health "challenges" between birth and 6 years old. There were moments when I was up all night; sleep deprived and even a little scared. But, the choices we made and how we dealt with those moments made a huge difference in the health of our children and the outcomes.

Life is hard enough with healthy children! I do not know what it is like to have a child who is always ill, suffering with asthma, severe food allergies on medications and always at the doctor's office, maybe with depression and anxiety, poor self esteem and emotional problems, learning problems, angry or suffers with autism or diabetes. I grieve when I meet parents who are challenged everyday with sick children who are always in pain or suffering and need constant medical care. I count my blessings that we were exposed to a different way and learned what to avoid before having our first daughter, Renee in 1980.

Our children were really healthy compared to most children and because of that, I am dedicated to sharing what we did that I believe made the huge difference. That is my motivation and my calling: I believe all children should have the opportunity to express their God-given health potential and what we do as parents will determine that outcome! Every decision we make will impact their life, some more than others."

Mary Tocco, Independent Vaccine Investigator, Public Educator, Natural Healthcare Advocate, www.childhoodshots.com, radio program called Healing Our World (RepublicBroadcasting.org)

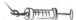

"Our second son, Jordan, was born on July 2, 1995. Another joyous day for my wife and myself. We had even more reason to celebrate because unlike our first son born 18 months earlier, Jordan was born without incident and was perfect in every way. In an extreme contrast to this, our first born had severe meconium aspiration after 33 hours of labor and was whisked away by a crash team as soon as he was delivered. Thankfully, after 3 intense weeks in the NICU he survived and as I write this, we are preparing for his high school graduation.

I am a Doctor of Chiropractic and among other things, I am opposed to the assault on the immune system known as vaccination. My wife and I had a birth plan as well as a life plan for our children to keep them healthy with a robust immune and nervous system. Then, the unthinkable happened.

At around 15 months of age, we were at a family reunion and my aunt, a teacher, mentioned that Jordan did not seem quite right. He had no language at all. Of course, I took offense and brushed it off as a meddling, know-it-all relative. However, at

17 months of age, we knew there was reason for concern. So began our journey of hop scotching the US and Canada to find a cure or at least help. When Autism was suggested, I angrily denied it because my son was not vaccinated. That sort of thing only happens to those that give in to the medical system and allow all of that poison to be injected into their children's body. It must be something more. After seeing some of the foremost authorities on childhood development, including Stanley Greenspan, and a host of experts in the medical, chiropractic and alternative fields, we accepted Jordan's faith.

Unlike other Autistic children, Jordan never had language nor developed with the milestones you hear of and then suddenly lost everything. His issues were more than the simple turning of a switch. Some things matched the true Autistic spectrum and others did not. Major bowel issues (constant diarrhea like applesauce), stammering, lack of eye contact, food aversions, social disconnect, repetitive behavior, fascination with videos, poor response to pain and other common findings were there. But why him? Why us? We did everything right and our baby is locked in his own world. I began to make calls and inquire. During my search, I found other chiropractors that also had unvaccinated, Autistic children. Wow - it is not just me.

We arranged to have a MRI performed of his brain which answered part of our questions. The results demonstrated a partially unmyelinated brain. What could have caused this? As I read and researched, I found out that this is what happens to the nervous system with, among other things, mercury poisoning.

On reflection, I recalled that during the crisis of our first born, my wife (who was exhausted and overwhelmed), was literally separated from me and taken into a separate room. Here, she was coerced against our birth plan to receive a Rhogam shot due to the Rh factor incompatibility between her and my son (O- vs. B+). She recalls having no fight left in her and at that point, did not care about anything but our son struggling for his life. At that time, in the mid-1990s, this vaccine was loaded with mercury. It has always been my suspicion that high mercury levels in her body caused Jordan's brain and nervous system to under-develop especially since we conceived only 9 months after our first was born.

Perhaps there is a genetic factor making one more susceptible to mercury poisoning. Perhaps there is a link to maternal toxicity and neonatal development. I know everything has a cause, and at this point in time with no other answers and a soon to be 17 year old son that can not talk, communicate and needs 24/7 care, my beliefs can only lead me to believe that the Rhogam shot my wife received caused Jordan's Autism. So while he himself never received any drugs or shots throughout his life, he remains a mystery with, in my opinion, only one logical explanation."

"I am not sure what caused my son's autism, but autistic he IS! It's a heart wrenching disease. He is completely unvaxed as we stopped vaxing 10 years ago. However, I did receive the Rhogam shot while pregnant and that has Thimerasol in it. In addition, he got antibiotics through breast milk at 2 months, then he received ABX at 13 months for a fever, which caused a febrile seizure.

He started regressing after that and at age 2 was diagnosed with autism. He is now 6. He does not speak really. He can say Mama but does not always discriminate when and he says some sounds. He sometimes follows directions, like "sit"; he pretty much is a 6-year-old body and a 1-year-old communication ability.

When he was diagnosed, we replaced all chemical cleaners with natural cleaners like Shaklee's basic H, orange peel citrus cleaners. We got rid of our aluminum-anodized pans and replaced them with stainless steel, we stopped warming up foods in plastics.

We still do microwave popcorn and I have not been able to do a GF diet yet but that is the next step. I don't believe he'll ever live an independent life. He is not potty trained though it is coming along slowly at preschool.

Asperger's runs in our family and I believe the RX products aided in triggering his autism."

"Before we had our firstborn we were unsure whether we wanted to vaccinate or not. We were caught in the middle. Our intuition was telling us something wasn't right and our society was telling us we had to do it. We realized our doubts would only turn into clear decisions with education and knowledge. So we started with a very educational science based video by Dr. Tenpenney. It was extremely informative and that video really opened my eyes to corporate greed and power and the influence all these pharmaceutical companies have, unfortunately and unbelievably even at the sacrifice of our children. We started to watch more videos and read books by Barbara Loe Fisher. What really sealed our decision was when we read about the independent study that was done in West Coast, USA, (generation something?) that basically showed the health and other mental factors of children over certain amount of years and the major differences between vaccinated and unvaccinated children. We truly came to the conclusion that the risks definitely don't outweigh the benefits (if any) of vaccination.

So we were now armed with enough knowledge to make the right decision for our child. And we are so happy that we made that decision.

Our firstborn is now 6 years old and our second-born is 3 years old. Our children are amazingly healthy and have built up their own immunity naturally. Through proper diet, love, and we believe not introducing toxic chemicals into their bloodstream our children have never taken a pharmaceutical drug and have never gotten a major sickness. We constantly see children around us getting really sick all the time. We see high fevers, ear aches, chronic coughs, extreme virus symptoms, hospitalizations, and we never experienced any of that with our children. And this extreme sickness seems very normal in our society. Our children will catch a cold, and their symptoms will include a bit of a runny nose and congestion, and it will totally go away within 24 to 48 hours with natural care. We see the difference firsthand between our children and children around us that are being vaccinated. We are hopeful that enough parents become informed where one day the mainstream will not be vaccinating but helping their child build natural immunities to live healthy long lives."

"We have four children, two of which have not been vaccinated at all, and the older two underwent vaccines during the first two years of life. After a couple of bad reactions with my second infant, we began reading more and more about vaccines and realized something is not right with this approach. There just seemed to be too many hazardous chemicals and unnecessary things going into my very new little one. We are so careful of infants in all other ways, making sure we hold them right, feed them the right thing, etc., except when it comes to the vaccine schedule! WOW!

Our two youngest, now 4 and almost 2 have traveled the world without a single vaccine. We lived in Nepal and India for the past 6 years with no problems. They are some of the healthiest children I know, I think because I nursed them all for over a year, gave lots of fermented foods, lots of fruits and veggies, not very much sugar. Their immune systems are very strong. My first son has had many issues growing up, and he has been the most vaccinated. Issues include ADHD type symptoms, nervousness, ear infections (of course we had him drinking a lot of pasteurized milk before we knew that we shouldn't), and a couple of severe headaches that have lasted an entire day. Other than my first son, none of my children have used antibiotics, and non have ever contracted any kind of disease. We are a happy vaccine free family, putting their trust in God's wisdom of eating and taking care of our bodies with REAL foods and REAL sunshine!"

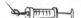

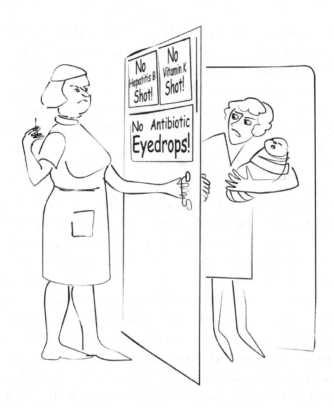

"When I became pregnant with my daughter, I started researching. The research was prompted by my neighbor who had three children. Her first child was fully vaccinated and had an array of health, disciplinary and behavioral issues. Her second child was partially vaccinated until 6 months when the vaccines caused a life threatening respiratory illness. She was told her son would never recover from the illness and probably die from it before the age of 5. She stopped vaccinating him, started him on a vaccine detox program and soon he was cleared of the illness. Her third child, a girl, is completely shot-free and has never been sick.

She told me her story and I looked back on my life as a vaccinated child. I was constantly sick and would develop severe fevers after vaccination, most often coming down with strep throat or other illnesses shortly after being vaccinated. I was diagnosed with an immune disorder very early in life and mysteriously developed a thyroid disorder months after being vaccinated with the Hep. A shot as a teen. My sister was no different and developed a "mysterious" leg tingling and fainting problem, coincidentally after three rounds of the HPV vaccine. Her symptoms became more severe with each dose but no doctor or specialist would admit a link to the vaccine. Ironically we were both encouraged to keep up to date on our shots because of our immune problems!

My mother had problems as a child as well. She cannot receive a flu shot because of the deadly side effects she suffers. With all of this in front of me, I was still being told that my child would surely die without vaccines and that she was at a higher risk of infection because the immune disorders could be hereditary. It was imperative that she receive vaccines because of my medical history. My neighbor gave me a book on vaccination, written by a doctor who is frowned upon in the medical community. The book was heavily referenced with documents from our own government and the pharmaceutical companies themselves. I quickly realized that vaccines possibly do not protect against disease at all and no one has any idea which child's immune system will trigger a response to vaccines and which child will become permanently brain damaged or immune suppressed! No one truly knows if vaccines cause cancer, SIDS, or autism. In fact, many studies point to vaccines as the cause!

Some are surprised to hear that I was still on the fence at this point. With so many doctors threatening that my child would surely die a horrible death of whooping cough or be permanently damaged by polio, how could I not pay attention to their fear mongering and bullying? I was told that mothers who neglect their children and are careless about their lives don't vaccinate. I was told my child would not be allowed in public school and could possibly be taken away from me for my carelessness. So I kept researching. How could I live in a free country that does not allow me to have a choice in the uncertainty that is injected into my precious little infant's helpless body?

I was 9 months pregnant with my daughter when my dog died as a reaction to a rabies shot. Within hours of being injected he started to drool and twitch. Within days he was bumping into things and could not turn his head to the left. After a week he would not eat or drink, was foaming at the mouth from dehydration and whimpering in pain. If he stood up, he could not keep himself from spinning in circles to the right. His symptoms became so severe, so quickly, and I remember holding him still to feed him water from my hand. He whimpered and struggled for every last drop. He knew he was dying and cuddled with me at night. In just one week, I was back at the veterinary office four times to put him on antibiotics and other medications. The doctors told me it was a random virus that had crossed the blood brain barrier and it was not a result of the rabies vaccine that he had received hours before the start of his symptoms. I had done my research. Viruses don't just cross the blood brain barrier and house dogs don't just come down with debilitating diseases. We put him down and I knew that I had witnessed first hand what a vaccine can do to a body.

I was still scared but I posted signs on my delivery room door that my infant was not to have the vitamin k shot, the Hep. B shot or antibiotic eye drops. I even got into a verbal fight with a nurse, who had needle in hand, who told me that my baby girl would die within a few days if she did not get at least the vitamin k shot. I cried over my daughter's crib, thinking I had put her at risk to disease. I kept researching and became confident with my decision. My second child, a boy, came along and I did not vaccinate him either. Upon refusing the vitamin K shot, I was denied his circumcision. At his 1 week appointment, I had two doctors and a nurse corner me, with the vitamin k shot ready to be injected, telling me that my son would bleed to death if he was circumcised without the shot. I tried to compromise by allowing oral vitamin k but the doctors refused to write the prescription, stating that their licenses were on the line and the oral vitamin k was not effective enough to prevent him from bleeding to death because of my negligence. It didn't take me long to find another doctor who had been in practice for over 35 years and was willing to do the circumcision without vitamin k.

My children do not get sick. My daughter had swimmers ear for two days when she was 6 months old. My son had a fever of 101 degrees for one whole day when his front two teeth came in. If you call that sick, then what do you call the parents who have to deal with ER visits and ear infections every other month? It's been 4 years now and my children have somehow survived, THRIVED without vaccines. I truly believe that, given my medical history, if I had vaccinated my child, one of them would be permanently damaged or dead. I truly believe in my children's immune systems and I will spare nothing to protect them from vaccines! I will fight for my rights to protect their health and their lives. I hope I can spread the word to other potential victims of vaccination and I pray that vaccines will be outed in my lifetime."

"I am the mother of three unvaccinated children; a son age 7, a daughter age 10, and a son age 11. My husband and I made the educated choice not to vaccinate our children when they were babies. As I have been a vegan for 12 years, I also chose to remain a vegan during my pregnancies and had natural childbirth with all three children. The health of my children has always been my highest priority. During the toddler years, each one of my children experienced excellent health with no major illness that required a doctor's visit. Whenever they did get sick with fever or cold, their immune system was strong and illness was never prolonged. All three children have had regular dental visits since they were young; my oldest has never had a cavity, while the other two have only one cavity each.

While I home schooled them until two years ago, my children are now attending public elementary school. As my parental right to do so, I have waived all vaccine requirements for school attendance. I am now a single mother to my three children, and

I remain devoted to raising them in continued good health. As they grow into their pre-teen years, my oldest is no longer vegan, my daughter is now vegetarian, and my youngest remains vegan. Their entire life, I have educated my children on the importance of caring for their bodies, and I know that I have laid the foundation for them to make healthy choices when I am not around. Almost 12 years ago at the birth of my first child, I lovingly held him in my arms and felt that life was so precious. I knew then, I would do anything to keep him safe. For me, that meant the very first decision of many in my child's life, was to not vaccinate. I have never regretted it since."

"I have 3 children who are now 11, 8 and 5. I made the decision to not vaccinate because it ultimately comes down to trust, and frankly, I don't trust the government or the drug companies ("Big Pharma") they represent. I believe that the government uses vaccination as a cheaper option to containing infectious diseases rather than eliminating poverty, providing medical care to all, providing as many sick days and paid time off for families to nurse themselves and their sick children back to health and access to a truly healthy diet with unprocessed foods, grass fed meat and no sugar. Epidemiologically speaking, vaccines appear to work, but the problem is that researchers, doctors and other „experts" don't really know biologically what impact they have on the body. I will refuse to vaccinate until this information is known. And by this I mean research must be done and funded by an independent source, not by those who have a financial interest in the outcome.

My children are very healthy and never had antibiotics. But in spite of that, they do have a lot of food allergies. Gluten sensitivity, allergies to all grains, etc. We have a very low grain diet now, along with homeopathy, chiropractic and alternative allergy treatment. I feel like they are pretty healthy despite the food allergy thing. But the fact that they have food allergies, (chronic stomach aches, body aches, head aches, fatigue and some hyperactivity) I am even more convinced that not vaccinating them was the right decision for them. One of the best I ever made. Actually, my homeopath said that it was a good thing I never vaccinated my son because otherwise his problems would have been much worse. He had some anxiety and sensory issues as a young child. My second child had eczema and a chronic runny nose as well as some ear infections. She also had sensory issues in regards to wearing clothing and shoes. My third has no sensory but has the worst of the food allergy symptoms, suffering with chronic reflux. All of my children were breastfed for at least 2 years. So because I breastfed and didn't vaccinate, I expected that they wouldn't have such bad allergies. But I still stick by my decisions not to vaccinate."

"Honestly, I don't feel like I have that much to say about my unvaccinated children (3 and 8 years old). Their medical history is extremely boring. They are rarely ill and, if they do catch a cold, it doesn't last long. They have no developmental abnormalities (granted, I think they are very clever, but not abnormally so). They have great muscle tone, are active and agile, can focus on tasks... they don't have any problems that I have been able to identify... their childhoods have been blissfully uneventful as far as medical or health issues are concerned."

"My children were not vaccinated. Well, my older daughter was partially vaxed at 2, 3, 4 months with dt and polio, no pertussis. At the time I was working as a homeopath in the UK and was treating many children with chronic immune conditions, ear problems, eczema and asthma, etc. that I noted all seemed to come up after vaccines one way or the other. I decided to not vax anymore and am so glad I did. I was also trained as a biologist and have amassed over 20 years of research to back up my decision. Much is available now due to the internet but back then I relied on medical papers and things like the 'Informed Parent' a monthly parent newsletter and WDDTY, a British alternative publication.

Our family moved to countries a bit and it was made apparent to me the different rules in each country with no apparent rationale other than do what they say. I fought the docs all the way and was many times in tears coming out of physicals with my kids as I was made to feel, well, you know.

Anyway, I stuck to my ground and am glad to say they have all been treated homeopathically or with natural means whenever they were sick. They have never had an antibiotic or an allopathic medical intervention in their lives, except my son who broke his leg and had to be operated on. The nurse who took his medical details could not believe that a 14-year-old was as free from doctor's meddling as he was. She had never seen it before– we now live in the US.

They have no allergies, immune problems etc. Sure they get the odd cold but a couple of days rest and good food they are as right as rain. They are all physically very active in swimming, crew and other sports.

I believe the power of nature is far superior to any current medical fads."

"My daughter is 18 months old. She has never received a single vaccine. We have a history of autoimmune disease on both sides of the family. After doing much research I do not feel vaccination is the best option for my child. I go to a homeopathic pediatrician in Tampa, Dr. Berger, who respects my decision. His practice specializes in treating children who have autism and other behavioral disorders. He also treats children who have been hurt in some way by vaccinations and I can see this firsthand while in the waiting room of his office chatting with parents. In some cases he is able to reverse the side effects through specialized treatment.

My daughter is gorgeous and absolutely healthy as can be. I do everything I know through diet and lifestyle to keep her healthy. She gets 30 minutes of sun almost every day (as long as it is warm enough). I breast-fed her for 11 months. I limit the amount of sugar in her diet. We juice vegetables and she loves the taste. She gets lots of protein, omega-3's, and probiotics. If she catches a cold we have a first-signs-of-illness protocol recommended by her doctor (Vit. A, Zinc, Vit. C and Echinacea) rather than immediately running to the clinic for antibiotics. We use colloidal silver instead which is just as effective.

I realize the threat of getting sick is still a reality. However, I would much rather treat the illness than witness her living with the side effects of poisoning from a vaccine manufacturer that is more interested in fattening his/her pockets than they are in the well-being of my kid whom they will never ever meet.

I refuse to live with regret for a decision I know in my heart is NOT right for my family. They can bully someone else. I will not succumb to their pressure. I do not feel guilty for my decision. I feel like I am way more educated than most traditional doctors who only read what the drug manufacturers tell them to read. I have more at stake than they do. Therefore I do my research, I continually educate myself on these subjects and I continually reevaluate my decision based on new information. I've weighed my options and know I am making the right choice. I am meeting more and more parents who feel the same way I do. People are waking up!"

"My 13-year-old daughter is completely unvaccinated. She is very healthy, intelligent, creative, and well-adjusted. She is rarely ill, has never taken an antibiotic, and never had ear infections or other chronic infections as a baby. She does not take any prescribed medications, and usually only sees the doctor for an annual check-up. She scores well on her annual academic achievement tests, and even scores at the college level on the language and verbal portions of the test. She plays piano, draws well, writes short-stories and poetry, and was recently accepted by audition to train in the summer program of a major ballet company. I have not yet had her titer-tested, so I do not know which of the diseases our state commonly vaccinates children for she has acquired natural immunity to, but she did contract chicken pox last year, and so now has life-long immunity to that: immunity she will be able to pass on to her own children via placenta and breast milk. Her bout with chicken pox was uncomfortable, but uneventful and uncomplicated.

When I was pregnant with my daughter, I knew nothing about the controversy surrounding vaccination, and so right up until the last few weeks of my pregnancy, I had every intention of vaccinating her. Then a friend who didn't vaccinate her children asked me, "So are you planning to vaccinate her?" I replied, "Yes," and we dropped the subject. The following week, she asked me the same question. I replied the same as before, but suddenly a proverbial light went on in my head, and I thought, "There is something I don't know about vaccination." I began to research. By the time of her first well-baby check-up, I had learned just enough to know that I needed to know more, and that once I vaccinated her, I could never take it back. So I decided to delay indefinitely until I felt confident in myself about what decision I would make. Thirteen years later, I am still avidly following vaccine issues, and have purchased and read several excellent books on the subject of vaccination. Diseases are real, and so are vaccine injuries. There are no guarantees, but I feel that I have made the best decision I can with the information available to me."

"Mother of an unvaccinated 12 year old son. I was always interested in being healthy and taking care of myself, so once I found out I was pregnant I was on a mission to raising a very healthy child from the moment of conception. I researched the pros and cons of vaccination and I had no doubt in my mind and heart that I was not going to subject my child to the Russian roulette.

He is a gorgeous healthy, well balanced kid. I know I made the right choice and I have no regrets whatsoever. I will always support people to have a choice and to be educated about vaccinations. I wish more people would educate themselves before exposing their kids.

I'm so happy I took the time and had the guts to say no."

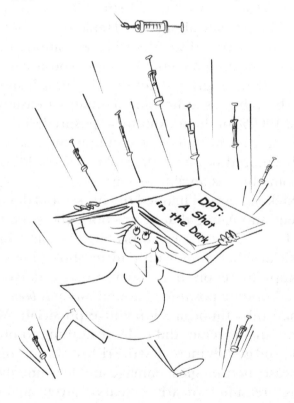

"My unvaccinated son, Nikolai, is now 13 years old - born in 1999. While I was still pregnant with Nick, by the grace of God, a friend handed a book called, 'A Shot in the Dark'. Written by Harris Coulter and Barbara Joe Fisher, it offers an extensive history on the

American blanket vaccine program, and the fallout in individual lives.

This introduction to the *'vaccine controversy'* was explosive for me, and timely. It provoked me to read extensively on the subject. With a pending birth to think about, and the life of my child hanging in the balance – I wanted to know the truth, although I found it impossible to get anything but obviously rote information from mainstream outlets like newspapers, magazines, or doctor's offices. So I put the time in to dig more deeply. Ultimately I read 25 books and hundreds of articles.

Then just before I gave birth, I stumbled across a statement made by Dr. Bob Sears about the Hepatitis B shot. Dr. Sears pointed out that the American Medical Association's own web site gives an infant's maximum recommended exposure to Aluminum Hydroxide as '25 micrograms'. Yet the Hepatitis B shot routinely given to newborn babies in hospitals contains an astonishing 250 micrograms! 1000% of the maximum exposure level!

In other words, not only is common-medical-sense being outrageously ignored but it doesn't take a whole lot of sleuthing to see that something is terribly wrong.

Before Nick was born, I handed the nurses and doctors a 'Birth Request Sheet' stipulating that he was not to be given any shots at all (in case I was out of it!) From his birthday on, I have worked with pediatricians that comply with my no-shots philosophy.

I am happy to report that I never had a doctor refuse us services based on our position. Though *had this been an issue*, I'd have searched till I found a cooperative physician. My research convinced me that vaccines did little or nothing to prevent short term disease, and greatly increased the risk of chronic disease, auto-immune disease, neurological damage and learning disabilities!

Nick was breast-fed (nearly 3 years), given an organic and healthy diet, and - as much as possible - we avoided processed foods, sodas, white sugar, antibiotics and even over the counter medicines. We let Nick play out of doors, in the mud, with puppies licking his face and get a typical exposure to bugs, nicks and bruises.

Nick did contract typical childhood illnesses including measles, mumps, chicken pox and a host of stuffy noses and simply got over them. I did not run to the doctor or even buy over the counter medicine to suppress his symptoms when Nick got sick, with the exception of some baby Tylenol for high fevers. By permitting him to be/get sick and spend the time recovering naturally, Nick developed the stellar immune system that I believe is the heritage of most children.

The upshot is that in 13 years Nick is the healthiest child we know. He has NEVER had an ear infection. He has no allergies, no learning disabilities, and at this writing Nick has not been sick at all since he was 7 years old! He can be in a room full of sick kids with runny noses, flu, strep throat - you name it - and not contract *anything*. Thanks to these philosophies, Nick has been permitted to achieve his personal best physically and academically. He bicycles, plays soccer, football and he is already strong enough to pick his mom up and carry her (you'd be impressed if you knew my weight)!

In public school Nick has been in advanced classes for years. This year for example, he's in 7th grade but taking 9th grade Algebra. With all my heart I believe Nick's good success is due to good food, a positive environment based on the love of God, the omission of pharmaceutical intervention and our permitting him to develop a natural and powerful immune system.

By way of contrast, my brother gave his daughter (one year older than Nick) a full schedule of vaccines as was recommended by their pediatrician. Today my niece has severe allergies, reacts to every little bug bite with terrible rashes, and gets sick all the time. When she visits, we have to be very careful about what she eats, and as a result she is unable to eat many healthy foods, exacerbating the cycle of un-wellness.

It has become my personal conviction that the federal government should not be in the business of practicing medicine. Too many children have been permanently harmed by the federal program of blanket vaccinations. I was astonished to discover that the eradication of many modern diseases arrived well before a vaccine had been developed for them. And that recorded outbreaks of disease have been documented as a result of administration of a vaccine, rather than the lack of it.

Finally, I will say, that here in the US I have never had the least difficulty registering my unvaccinated child for public school, private schools or camps. As a result of parental pressure in the wake of protracted damage, each of our 50 states takes any one of 3 waivers, be it philosophical, medical or religious. Anyone needs simply to research their state's laws, and take a firm stand (or move). I will never, ever, regret my decision to become an informed parent, and stand by my principles these 13 years now. I have a healthy happy child to show for that.

PS. I am 55 and have also not been sick more than a bad cold in Nick's lifetime. But then, I too steadfastly refuse all shots."

Victoria Jean Christine Bingham, Alexandria Virginia, vjcbok@bfresco.com

"All 3 of my children are unvaccinated. My daughter is almost 6, my oldest son is 4, and I have a newborn that is 6 weeks old. My oldest two play in dirt all day, they don't „sanitize" their hands, and they are two of the healthiest kids that I know! They have never been sick for more than 12 hours. And the times that they HAVE been sick I can count on my hand (between all 3 kids even). I think there has been about 4 times today. Probably 2 per each kid (none for the newborn). It amazes me (yet it doesn't really because it just makes SENSE!)...

As far as not vaccinating goes it just made sense to not vaccinate! My kids receive all their immunities from my breast milk and as far as being healthy goes, it shows in the amount that they are sick! I am very grateful that I do not immunize as it is not needed!!! Thanks for allowing me to share this."

"4th Generation ~Unvaccinated~. Did 'unvaccinated' exist before then? My parents were curious folks, in their youth. But, once they had discovered how to maintain good health each new medical discovery or advancement didn't seem that ground-breaking, curious, or phenomenal. Health always seemed to return to a strong foundation of self-care.

Midwifery, Chiropractic, and holistic medicine became special to my parents. Each pursued careers in these fields.

As I grew up, they used herbs, tinctures, 'weeds' from the yard and mountain side, chiropractic care, acupressure, healthier diet choices, exercise, fresh air, and rest to maintain good health or to recover good health.

Not vaccinating my own children was a simple decision, because despite what we had heard all of our lives, I had had absolutely no life-threatening illness overtake me, under any circumstance. My siblings and I would be ill at times, just like everyone else, but we would recover from illness promptly. Our blood, bones, and bodies were very healthy. Not only was each medical care provider we had aware of it, we could literally feel that our bodies were healthy, too.

Nothing we practice is perfectly practiced. It is hard to access the healthiest food, water, and medicine all of the time. But, we do allow for natural illnesses to take their course. I am confident that each illness my parents, myself, and my children encounter will become a lifelong immunity that we are grateful for. We aren't afraid.

Now, Biological Engineering is a whole other matter - some of this does worry me. God Bless the health of each person in need that reads this - for generations to come."

"I just cannot trust the pharmaceutical corporations' agenda because clearly they are out solely for profit. I believe most of the employees and CEOs believe in their products, but when the products are tested thoroughly by unbiased research scientists who are not paid by the interest group, that research is the information that I heed. And I am a true believer in staying away from all additives, preservatives, GMOs and processed foods, and I am not concerned about the diseases they want to protect my child from. I chose not to vaccinate my daughter, now 19 1/2, and she had a mild case of chicken pox - no problem. I see kids who eat a lot of sugar, simple carbohydrates and processed foods have the worst cases. We have been to India and she has been to Ecuador and had no shots. She's fine. Her health is fabulous. Even when she gets sick or was sick as a kid, I just let the fever take its course - water, tea, rest and more rest (I did not send my kid to school sick or even with a slight fever or if she still felt weak) and then light organic foods.

I am very, very grateful I did not vaccinate my child and wish that others were better educated and had the courage to stand up to the brainwashing system. It is scary that Big Pharma is pressuring the government to take away the option of not immunizing for philosophical reasons. People need to know and have their rights!"

"I have two children, a 15-year-old boy and 13-year-old girl, both are unvaccinated. They are healthy, active, and social children. They go to school, have played on several different teams in sports, both took dance classes for several years and have lots of friends. They've only been on antibiotics a couple of times in their lives and have had no major illnesses. The fifteen-year-old is doing high school and college at the same time and has a 4.0 GPA. He's worked part time with his father on construction sites since he was 10. When he was 12 and playing outside he broke his foot in 3 places and it healed nicely. My thirteen-year-old is in middle school and takes dance classes now. She wants to be a chef.

Our family has traveled the country extensively over the years. We have visited Mexico and Canada as well. Our kids have never had any illnesses that vaccinations would have fixed, nor given anyone else an infectious disease.

I have been very pleased with the results and if I had it to do over again I would. My husband is in agreement with this also."

"My healthy son will be three in August 2012. He was breastfed until he was just over two years old. He has never had any vaccinations. He eats a diet of organic pasture-raised meats, organic eggs and vegetables and raw milk and milk products. He gets no processed foods or sugar (only raw honey and maple syrup). He is rarely sick. This past winter, he only had a few running noses and minor coughs, but never was in bed, feverish or otherwise ill. I exposed him in March to chicken pox by swapping spit on a stick with his cousin who was getting active sores. My son never contracted the disease. He is strong, agile and beautiful. He is verbally and socially advanced, and sweet as can be. We have our moments, but he rarely has anything like a tantrum."

"Before our first child was born, we made the firm decision to keep our children vaccine-free. Let it be known that it was met with opposition and hatred by an uneducated medical community and public. When our first son was born, he had had some trauma to his head from the birth process. When we refused the Vitamin K, we were told that he would suffer brain injury because he would not be able to stop the bleeding. We respectfully declined and when push came to shove, they admitted that he would be fine. Later on, the pediatrician threatened that if our child did not get vaccinated at the hospital, he would run the risk of dying from the measles or whooping cough.

Needless to say, our resolve for each subsequent child to remain vaccine-free strengthened. Today we have three beautiful, bright, mentally-aware children that have never had a medication or toxic vaccine in their bodies ever. They've never suffered from allergies, asthma, and have never had an illness last longer than a few hours. We know that the symptoms of illness (fever, cough, diarrhea, etc.) are actually the CURE to overcome illness. When they do start to express the symptoms, we honor and facilitate the healing, rather than try to cover up the symptoms.

Our children today get adjusted weekly, eat organically, and take vitamins. They are the fullest expression of health....just the way God intended."

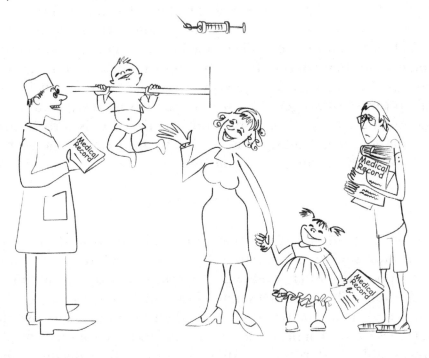

"I have three children, two of whom are not vaccinated. My daughter, Wynter, is three and she has a power house immune system. She has picked up a couple illnesses but nothing has ever lasted more than 12 hours and she has never had to be seen for it. She has fabulous focus and even learned to read many words before she was 2. My youngest son, Sterling, is 2 and has never been sick with anything. He is also focused and very strong, our gymnastics instructor said she has never witnessed a 2-year-old do a pull up before Sterling. Our doctor says these two have the thinnest files in the office! My first born Austin, now 17, was fully vaccinated. From 1995-2007 he had 24 vaccinations. He had severe chronic bronchitis as a baby, he still suffers from croup, he gets sick every season, and he has limited focus and little energy. I definitely can tell the differences in my children and wish I could go back in time and choose to say no with my first born as well."

"I am 50 years old and was never vaccinated. My children are now 14 and 15 and have not been vaccinated. Luckily for me, my mother was very curious and open to alternative health directions when she had her 5 children in the 1950s and 1960s. She chose to breastfeed all 5 of her babies when bottle feeding was not only the norm, but encouraged by physicians; she chose not to vaccinate her 5 babies because of her distrust and skepticism of the prevailing medical thoughts; she regularly visited her chiropractor. All of us children have grown up healthy, disease free, and without depression. We are all very physically active people and at ages 50-62, none of us are on any prescription medicines whatsoever (and by the way, we all see chiropractors, acupuncturists, and massage therapists as part of our healthcare routine). Thankfully, I was able to educate my husband when our babies were born about the "other" side of vaccination. He was willing to go along with my wishes and now that he has become educated, is an advocate against vaccination just like me. Doctors do not always know best. In fact, they often do harm. My unvaccinated children are now old enough to appreciate that their parents seek the whole truth about health issues and I feel confident they will continue to question and challenge the world they're living in.... seeking to find what makes the best sense for them.

Vaccine Free

It was easy for me to seek this direction for them because that's what I learned from my mom, bless her soul. By the way, my mom turns 89 next month and is still healthy as can be."

"My son is now 28 months old. I chose not to vaccinate after researching statistics, vaccine ingredients, and experiencing my friends' child's seizures directly following his first round of vaccinations. She is a nurse and has since decided not to vaccinate. I won't claim it's been a well received choice by friends, family, and opinionated strangers (especially with our current whooping cough „epidemic" in Washington) but I feel secure about my decision. My sons' health is great. I also won't claim any superpowers for him but I do see he has a strong immune system and bounces back quickly from any little sniffle he acquires. One of the vaccinated children at his school has just been diagnosed with whooping cough in the last month and we have yet to see any symptoms in him though they had been in constant contact. We have also taken him out of country without his vaccinations with modest precautions. The human body is a miraculous and beautifully running thing and yet we treat it like a broken machine unable to heal itself and adapt to diverse exposures. I feel he can make different decisions about his body when he's older if he so desires."

"My child has never been vaccinated; she is nearly 2 1/2. She is not only completely healthy but remains so whenever she is in a class with other children (who were vaccinated) that are ill. I feed her healthy, all organic foods and rotate the foods (all milks, grains, meats, oils, nuts especially) so she never repeats any food for at least one week. She eats a HUGE variety of foods and grains; never anything processed or refined. She has a terrific appetite and enjoys countless types of foods (eggplant being her favorite). My daughter is healthy - she has only had one cold since she has been alive and that was because a nanny coughed directly in her face (however my daughter recovered in 3 days, the nanny in 2 weeks!). My daughter is radiant - her face and hair shine so much so that others always mention it. My daughter is relaxed and happy - her mind is clear and she is always in a good mood since preservatives/chemicals are not "fuzzing" up her brain. My daughter is brilliant - with a clear mind and food that feeds her body and brain she is totally focused and though she is two, she speaks, acts and thinks like a 6-year-old, her doctors are always astounded by her and her grasp on language & concepts. My daughter is free - she is free from preservatives and animal DNA strands in immunizations, free from toxic foods that the FDA deems acceptable; she is free to be everything that she chooses to be rather that suffering what is thrust upon her by chemicals, preservatives, artificial ingredients and poison immunizations.

As a parent, it is my job to protect my child, I can not ever imagine willingly giving my child an immunization that can potentially damage my child. I don't care about statistics, I care about my child. If something only affects 1 in 100, well I only have 1 and that is all I worry about. Bravo to all parents who CHOOSE wisely for their children!"

"When I became pregnant with my daughter five years ago, although I had been through acupuncture school and had been around lots of natural-minded parents, I had not heard anything about the vaccine issue. I simply accepted the rhetoric that I had been fed for years as scientific truth: that vaccines alone were responsible for the decline of infectious disease mortality throughout the world. It wasn't until I had three or four parents tell me that they hadn't vaccinated their children that I began to think about the issue at all. My friend's children were bright, healthy children with radiant glows in their complexions. I didn't think much of it, but decided that it was at least worth looking into the other side of things. The more I began to find out, the more unsettled I began to feel with the idea of having my baby vaccinated. Story after story began surfacing of healthy babies falling into stupors and developing seizures after vaccines, and anecdotal evidence aside, I began to discover that there was almost NO credible research to support the effectiveness and safety of vaccines, and it was that more than anything else which solidified my resolve to prevent my baby from becoming a guinea pig at a tender age. It was beyond my comprehension that in spite of FDA regulations that all medications undergo double blind, placebo controlled trials, that most vaccines had never been tested in this way. In my naivety, I had always placed blind trust in our government to be the watchdog for public safety.

My daughter was born without painkillers with the help of a midwife who was a family friend, weighing 6 lbs, 5 ounces, and was amazing from the beginning. She was so alert that her father snapped a photo of her tiny hand clasping his glasses seconds after she had emerged from the birth canal. She slept peacefully in my room with me, as I had planned to breastfeed, and awakened only once or twice for a diaper change. Our first week at home was peaceful and idyllic, as she slept most of the time, and breastfeeding was going reasonably well. We arrived for our first pediatrician appointment a week later at Premier Pediatrics in Park Slope, Brooklyn, which was the office of the doctor who had assessed my daughter for her Apgar score, which was 9.

Everything went well, as the doctor weighed my daughter, and began chatting with me about how things were going, until we decided to present a question. "What about vaccination?" my daughter's father asked. "Were there any risks to it?" The doctor's face immediately fell, and he became almost angry. "You had really impressed me until now," he said, "but I hope you don't make a decision which will make me think less of you." Alex continued that we simply wanted some information about risks, and that we were trying to make an informed decision for our child. The doctor looked pointedly at us and put it very bluntly: "If you do not vaccinate your child, we will not continue to keep you on as patients." We left the office having felt that we were treated as criminals simply for asking for more information about vaccines.

Thankfully, I belonged to a parenting list server at the time, and there were many discussion threads pertaining to vaccination, and I was able to find several doctors in our area who allowed parents to choose whether or not to vaccinate their child. One of them happened to be a family friend of a distant relative of Alex's, as luck would have it, and he was able to take us on as patients. My daughter was very healthy her first year, and she had only one or two minor colds, with some congestion, that I treated with some pediatric Chinese herbs and a few sessions of eucalyptus steam by putting her in her car seat in the bathroom and turning on the shower so that the room would steam up. I put about ten drops of oil in the tub, and this seemed to help quite a bit. My daughter seemed surprisingly unaffected by the serial ear infections, unrelenting coughs, and bowel issues that seemed to plague other parents. She slept very well at night, and by the time she was two months old, was sleeping five to six hour stretches between midnight and 6 am, which thankfully, allowed me to rest. When she did wake up, I simply put her to my breast immediately, and after feeding she would fall again into a blissful slumber. She took her first steps around 11 months, and began speaking in full sentences by 14 months.

My son was born 18 months later, and laboring him was considerably less painful than with my daughter. I walked a few blocks to our local hospital and gave birth to him without painkillers or even IVs with the help of my midwife. Both of my children have been remarkably unaffected by any ailments except the occasional cold, and one bout of a bad stomach flu, which we were able to moderate the effects of with some Chinese herbs. Their development has been normal, and they were both verbal at an early age. My son's health was very good, and only suffered some constipation after he was given some soy based baby formula at 11 months old. After he began drinking regular milk, his bowel movements became normal again.

I didn't discuss the vaccination issue with most parents unless I became close to them. I had read all sorts of comments on the parenting list server about how vaccine dissenting parents were leeches who benefited from herd immunity without having to vaccinate their own children and about a doctor whose daughter seized after the DTP vaccine but he continued to vaccinate her anyway. In spite of all the negative commentary, there were also lots of positive discussions regarding non-vaccination, and I discovered activists like Dr. Palevsky who disseminate factual, medically based information regarding vaccine topics. I don't regret the decision I made, although I worried quite a bit about how I would feel if my daughter contracted something and the especially high risks given that we live in New York City, where lots of people are in close contact with each other. I strongly believe that my children benefited from the immune factors they received by breast feeding, and that their immune systems have become stronger by fighting infections naturally. I was lucky to have contact with some of my holistic parent friends from California, who also told me about child friendly homeopathic remedies (which thankfully, I did not need to use) in case of illnesses.

My children are now three and four years old, and are enrolled in preschool. I was able to get a vaccine exemption based on my personal beliefs, which involved writing a letter to the school administration, and having the letter notarized and signed by our pediatrician. My children did pick up a few colds from school, but are overall very healthy, and recover very quickly from fevers and coughs with the help of herbal syrups and tinctures from the local health food store. I continue to learn more about this topic though, and began to blog sporadically about parenting issues and herbal medicine. As a parent, I was firstly, lucky to have been clued in by other parents, and secondly, persistent enough to do hours of online research, and uncompromising enough to make sure my children got a waiver before entering school. It is certainly not EASY to refuse vaccines, and it certainly is not the socially acceptable thing to do, but when I look at my bright, responsive, amazing kids, I can't imagine doing anything differently."

Marie Sepich LAc, http://bohemia78.blogspot.com

"My son was born in 2004. I feel so grateful that I had the exposure to the information that I did. Personally, I had been vaccinated as a child and had even a decade earlier received a tetanus vaccine. However, shortly before my son's birth, I became a student at a natural health school. Shortly after his birth, I became a student at yet another natural health school for my second degree. In both of these schools the power of prevention of illness in the form of vital nutrition, organic and whole food that is unprocessed as well as time in nature with the sun and the fresh air…exercise, play for children, etc.…were the main building blocks to health.

On the other hand, I learned that there were many toxins including formaldehyde and mercury, not to mention other ingredients of a very questionable nature, in vaccines. I learned that time and time again, when there were mass vaccine programs, there were also mass epidemics of the very disease that was vaccinated against. I learned that in most cases, many diseases had begun to decline well before the vaccine was introduced and this occurred due to improved nutrition and hygiene. Lastly, I learned that most sadly, many children had been permanently injured and or killed from being vaccinated and that the entire affair was a bit like Russian roulette.

For diseases such as chicken pox and the measles and mumps, not getting a vaccine was very easy to decide. I understood the basics of how to work with these illnesses naturally to minimize discomfort and appreciated that going through them my son would in most cases acquire a genuine immunity. The tetanus shot was the last one that I considered to get or not. It was the book,

How to create a book about unvaccinated children.
A recipe for beginners.

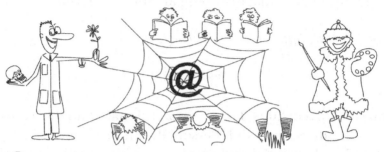

1. A homeopath from Switzerland, an artist from Siberia and internet users from around the world.

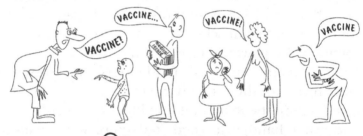

2. Observing the side effects of vaccines

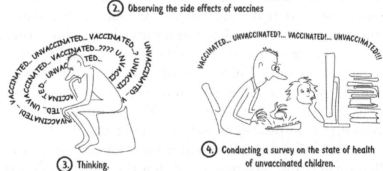

3. Thinking.

4. Conducting a survey on the state of health of unvaccinated children.

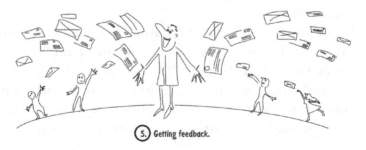

5. Getting feedback.

USA

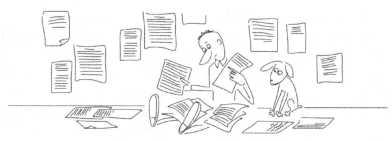

6. Selecting the most interesting stories.

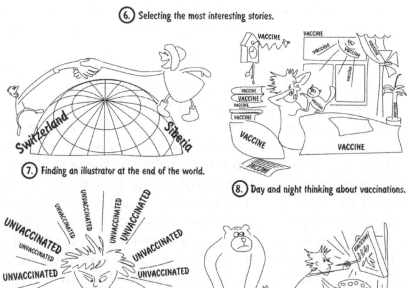

7. Finding an illustrator at the end of the world.

8. Day and night thinking about vaccinations.

9. Surviving the throes of creation.

10. Drawing.

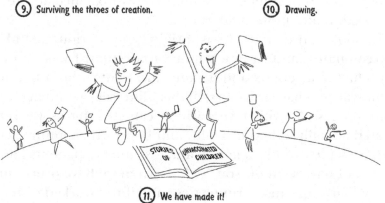

11. We have made it!

How to Raise a Healthy Child, in spite of Your Doctor, by Robert Mendelson, that helped to make my decision. Dr. Mendelson had not only been a pediatrician for over twenty years, he was a professor in the field. He noted that each year the page with the side effects of the tetanus vaccine kept getting longer and longer. At the same time as reading this, I learned that one could soak the affected area with Epsom salts and then cover with the blood cleansing herb Plantain, and that this was helpful in puncture wounds. In fact, my teacher had helped reverse serious blood poisoning situations with this very treatment.

Now eight years later, I have learned even more. I have learned that Louis Pasteur had said that we must protect ourselves from invaders such as bacteria. Yet, on his death bed, he changed this statement and instead agreed with his rival and peer Antoine Bechamp, that health was determined by the state of one's inner terrain. In a nutshell, we protect ourselves by being healthy....To me injecting formaldehyde and viruses and bacteria directly into the bloodstream seems to be the last thing that will build health.

Thus, I have opted to raise my son in what I consider a healthy way. I feed him whole food, which is raised organically....much actually by our family. We spend a great deal of time outside. We do not have a TV and keep movie watching to a very low number, opting to play games and read together. We work on healthy expression for a sound emotional life (stress is one of the main causes of impaired immunity). We balance activity with introspection and more quiet time.

My son is thriving. He is bright and curious....kind and compassionate....and so much more aware than I was at his age. He has had chickenpox and it came and went without that much irritation at all. I have learned that this "illnesses" are great cleaners of our bodies. As with fevers which can as long as we remain hydrated actually aide our health and boost our immune activity. So we drink juices and eat lightly, and rest and are patient. The only times that I have seen my son "sick" is when we have overindulged in dairy. This can cause a runny nose and if not worked with in the beginning grow into a cough. This is the only type of "illness" that my son has ever had. Because I see our role in this, I do not see it as sickness. I truly believe that we are meant to be healthy and well. We are meant to be vibrant free of this medical intervention. This is normal and natural. It is only when we deprive our bodies of the natural that our bodies tell us that this is not adequate for us.

Some of the new legislation concerns me. In California, a school was coming door to door and vaccinating children. Many well thinking parents do not know this alternative perspective and also do not know their legal rights. Almost every state has waivers for vaccines. You must see what your particular state says. Some states have philosophical waivers, while others are medical or religious.

Also, it was hard around some of my relatives. My father-in-law, a lawyer, flat out told me that I better not hurt his grandson. He refused to read the stacks of books that I had from school. I had to trust that I was doing the right thing.

To do this, it is imperative to be educated. A fantastic book that is full of documentation and true statistics is Vaccines....Are They Really Safe and Effective, by Neil Z. Miller. Excellent information. I also highly recommend learning natural ways of promoting health as well as dealing with "illness"."

"I am the mother of a 9-year-old girl and 11-year-old boy. My boy had his first round of shots when he was 1 1/2 years old. Then we took a trip to Texas to visit a very good friend who has two children damaged by vaccines (MMR). She questioned me about WHY I was vaccinating. Funny, as I really never thought about it before our conversation. It was just something that I was „supposed" to do. Well, I refused ALL vaccines from that moment on. My oldest attended kindergarden (public school) for one year and we have home-schooled ever since. We like to travel a lot. Usually by sailboat to different countries and have never had a problem with any sicknesses. My kids go to the doctor once a year just to get re-acquainted with our doctor. They really don't get sick. If they do get a touch of a cold it goes away very quickly. I have had to really „stand my ground" with a few doctors as they can be very intimidating at times. We must remember that here in the USA we still live in a free country, at least for now.

They are sharp, fast thinking children that have NO problem just sitting and relaxing on a sailboat for LONG periods of time. No hyperactivity anymore than a „normal" child and absolutely NO allergies which I think is the biggest problem with vaccines as well as flu shots given to children, pregnant women...and the elderly with aging brains. Remember to THINK TWICE."

"First a bit of history. My oldest daughter was completely vaccinated until the age of five. My second received two vaccinations (Polio and Hib) and the youngest two haven't had any. So I have experience with the health of both vaccinated and unvaccinated children to compare. The oldest gets ill the most often and it always hits her the hardest. Our middle daughter received a few vaccinations and while I find her health to be MUCH better than the oldest, she does have some asthma/bronchial issues that are mild. Both of the unvaccinated daughters handle their illnesses very well.

An example I would give is of her (4 year old) having the stomach "flu" that was going around the house. While my vaccinated child was passed out on the couch only semi-conscious, she was running around playing. Then she would stop to vomit, have a quick recovery cuddle and be back to running around a few minutes later. When she had chicken pox, it didn't itch and she did not have pain or other complaints. Maybe a very mild fever, but no real cold even. I've been more sick with a head cold than she was for Chicken Pox! Both the partially vaccinated and other unvaccinated child had the same experience (at different times) with getting Chicken Pox. They've all had Fifth Disease and

Hand Foot and Mouth as well. Never any complications or even trips to the doctor needed. Just rest and a bit of time. However, the younger ones always get much less ill and for a much shorter period of time than my vaccinated oldest girl. None of the two who weren't vaccinated have ever even needed an antibiotic. They have no allergies, no asthma, no major illnesses and not a single ear infection among them. My oldest had chronic ear infections that eventually required a tube, so it was great not to deal with those issues again. Usually none of them see the doctor during any given year unless it's a well visit check."

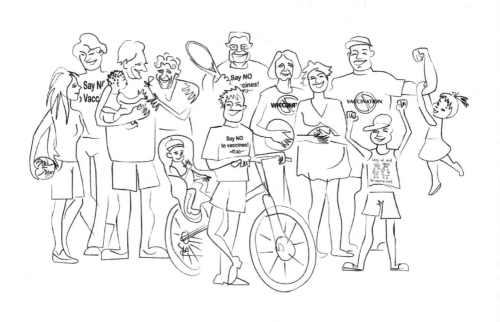

Canada

"We are the parents of six happy healthy children, now the fourth living generation of unvaccinated individuals. My grandparents, now in their 80's, have been hardworking, healthy, active people and still have a great zest for and interest in life; they live on their own and are alert and able, still gardening, and traveling, and enjoying their great grandchildren. Our parents are in their 50's and 60's, also unvaccinated, hardworking individuals; always enjoyed good health, and pursuing good lifestyle choices for their families. We are in our 30's and try also to maintain a healthy, active, un-medicated lifestyle. We have enjoyed healthy pregnancies and smooth, quick, un-medicated deliveries, never had issues with postpartum trouble, or behavioral difficulties with any of our children.

We do believe God is the giver of good health, but that the choices we make do affect that health. We live in a large community where there are lots of people who do not vaccinate, and I do not know anyone who has autism, etc. or any of the other common maladies of the day. We both have antibodies from when we went through measles, etc. as kids, and have had relatively easy journeys through the chicken pox, mumps, and whooping cough with our own. Having had the background of not vaccinating made the decision easy for us, yet we did do a lot of research about it when we had our first child. While we do not pretend to have all the answers, we are glad we have stuck with our original decision to not vaccinate, and we hope that many more are stimulated to do the same!"

"My son is a healthy 2.5-year-old. Both I and his father were vaccinated but when it came time to decide what we wanted for him, we decided to do some intense research. Having gone to school for training as a Holistic Health Care Practitioner, I am well versed in the amount of toxins that exist in products that are marketed to us as being "ok". The evidence on either side of the argument cannot discredit the toxins that are present in our vaccines and the separate medical research of what each of those toxins does to the human body. We simply decided this was not something we wanted to expose our son to. That being said, we do other things to make sure his body and immune system are working the way they should. I sneak organic veggies into every meal I can and limit the amount of processed foods he's given (at least at home because we can't live in a bubble). When he gets a cold, I use the appropriate herbs, essential oils and vitamins and minerals to strengthen his system further. If he gets a fever, I monitor it but never bring it down with over-the-counter medicines (at the very least for the first day or so) and he fights off the virus/infection very effectively. We see a ND as his primary care provider and also have open discussions with the family MD as to what diseases and illnesses are currently prevalent in our area that are deadly to a healthy child (none - covered in the government vax program).

It would be irresponsible to just "not vaccinate" your kids and ignore the fact that their developing bodies need to be supported to build strong immune systems. We are aware of the symptoms of serious illness and are very hands-on when it comes to his health. He even asks for his own vitamins if I happen to forget. Overall, my son is a happy, healthy, dirt-eating, bug-loving little boy. He meets or exceeds all "milestones" for his age group and still enjoys all the things a "normal" kid does.

Life is full of risks and choices - and we all have to live with the choices we make. What I think it comes down to (for me anyways) at the end of the day was this: If I vaccinated my son and a serious complication arose as a result, would I be able to live with myself?

OR - If I don't vaccinate him and he contracts a life-threatening (or worse) illness as a result, would I be able to live with the consequences? The thing is there are 2 guarantees in life: 1. you will die some day; and 2. life is unpredictable. Because of those guarantees, there was only one choice for me. Not vaccinating and taking the more "natural" approach to health is our lifestyle. Injecting harmful toxins into an infant to maybe "protect" against a few of the MANY "what-ifs" in life was not a risk I was willing to take. It's truly up to the parent(s) to be comfortable with their choice - either way - as they have to live with their child and the choices they make for them."

"Our son is 6 1/2 years old. Before he was born we researched vaccinations and came to a decision that we would not vaccinate our child - for many reasons. I have suffered from severe asthma, allergies and eczema my whole life. Knowing the hereditary traits of my health I knew that my child would probably have some of the same health issues. We didn't want to tax his system even more with vaccinations. The research always quoted scenarios from the 1800's and I didn't find that relevant to today's advancements in hygiene and medicine. I thought the degree of rareness of extreme symptoms did not justify the possible side effects from any vaccine. The autism link was another reason for us.

When we had our son we had a plan of what we wanted like no Vitamin K, no antibiotics, keep him connected to the placenta as long as possible etc...Well we all know that it doesn't go the way you plan. An emergency C-section happened and that changed the whole plan. The doctors told us that he needed to be put on antibiotics for a high white blood cell count. Vitamin K happened and the eye drops. But all was well. At the end another doctor came in and said that all new babies have a high white blood cell counts and we were furious at the outright lie that had been told by the first doctor.

Things have been in our control since then. When I told our family doctor that we would not be vaccinating our son he laughed at me mildly and said "Good luck getting him into school". Scare tactic that was completely not true. There was no problem with putting him into school nor have there been any problems with him being unvaccinated. The only problem was when he was younger, every time he got sick I would go on the computer and research again worrying that he had contracted something bad. Every time I did this it validated our decision.

So I would like to say... (knock on wood)...that our son is very healthy and strong. He gets sick but gets over it quickly. Now that he has gone through Kindergarten and most of grade one he has developed his immune system and seems healthier than ever. He rolls around in the dirt and even eats snow and plays at playgrounds with lots of germs! He has had eczema mildly since he was young but nothing like his mom (thankfully). He was a calm baby who slept well and wasn't very cranky. I've seen many vaccinated babies become very cranky, colicky and uncomfortable after their first injection. Just my observation. My sister is a nurse, actually a labor and delivery nurse and she couldn't understand why we had made this decision. Even with her education of the body she was tainted with western medicine's mindset. She had never even researched vaccines. Her daughter was one of those babies that became very cranky and unsettled after her vaccination. It may not have been directly after, a few weeks or a month but something had changed.

So we won't travel to certain countries that are more prone to some diseases. It has been worth it. I don't regret our decision. I just don't talk about it openly unless I am in the right crowd. It's a hot topic."

"We have five children currently ranging in ages 13 - 24. When our oldest son was born (24 years ago) we did not feel comfortable with vaccination. A cousin of mine recently had vaccinated her

3-month old daughter who developed severe seizures within 24 hours. There was no question that the vaccine she received had much to do with her seizures. This happened in 1988. At that time there was not much information available as to the safety of vaccines and no internet. Plus nobody else seemed concerned about this issue. No one was talking about it and there were no support or information groups to join. However we decided our baby's health was too important to blindly follow the status quo and the pressures of the public without at least doing some of our own research first so we could make our own educated decision. We did find some really good books available and which helped us to strengthen our convictions that vaccination was not a good idea. One important thing we learned was that vaccines contained harmful chemicals and toxins which could leave a child's immune and nervous system severely damaged. But even more importantly we learned that vaccination is not immunity, and by pumping "artificial immunizations" into our child's body we were risking damaging our child's naturally-designed immune system. These were risks we were not willing to take. It was a case of "the risk of vaccination being worse than the disease they were supposed to protect from."

Since that decision almost 25 years ago none of our children have been vaccinated. All of them are in excellent health and of healthy weight. Yes, they have had to deal with some minor viral and bacterial infections over the years such as respiratory and intestinal infections. But these have actually helped to strengthen their immune system the way their body was designed to. They always recovered 100% without the use of any medications, antibiotics, etc. Their healthy immune systems have allowed them to get through childhood without any of the common childhood illnesses such as throat infections, ear infections, allergies, asthma, eczema, digestive problems, etc. We have never seen any of these problems in our family. Our children have been 100% unvaccinated and unmedicated in the last 24 years. I should also mention that we do not follow the "normal" medical model. We have not had a family medical doctor in the past 20 years, instead opting to use naturopaths and chiropractors to stay healthy along with good nutrition and exercise.

Looking back we are 100% confident that we made the right decision not to vaccinate our children. It was our gift to them. Their robust health and the absence of illness speak for themselves. And we are thankful that our children plan to follow in our footsteps when they have families of their own."

"Vaccination Free 18 Years Later. I am one of those parents who has chosen not to vaccinate their children. I won't go into great detail with all of the reasons for this decision, but I will tell you that I do believe in the inherent power of the body to heal itself, especially when we get out of its way. I am writing this column to tell you how this has all worked out, eighteen years later.

I have two daughters, now age 18 and 17, and I made the decision not to vaccinate them after spending quite a bit of time and energy studying both sides of the story. I am grateful to have been aware that I even had a choice. I have to send blessings of gratitude to the families of the vaccine injured children who crossed my path years ago when I operated a local natural food store. They were brave enough to share their stories and help others like myself to realize that we do indeed have a choice in this matter. I believe that everything we experience, we experience for a reason, so I listened to what these families were telling me and I made the decision not to vaccinate. Shortly after making that decision fear started dogging me. The "what if?" thoughts and "how dare I be a bad mother" thoughts and the voice of the medical opinion started showing up for me to decide whether I was committing to my decision or giving in to fear. I breathed deeply, turned my attention deep within to access my wisdom, not just my intellectual programming, and found what was right for this situation.

Canada

Eighteen years later I am writing to report that my daughters are doing well. They have never been barred from any activity or opportunity because of their non-vaccinated status. They have traveled across the country, to different continents and environments and have remained well. They do get sick sometimes. I have observed their pattern of illness and recovery, it varies each time and between their individual constitutions, but it generally looks something like this: Day One feeling off balance; Day Two fever begins; Day Three fever increases; Day Three fever breaks and dissipates; Day Four to Day Ten or Eleven full symptoms of virus or infection appear and then dissipate; Day Twelve to Day Twenty One or so still not 100% but improving; Day Twenty Two+ generally feeling good and leaving the pattern of illness behind and new immunity developed.

I want to supply information to others who are making their decisions regarding vaccination by sharing our story. To vaccinate or not is a personal decision. Informed decisions help us to overcome making decisions just out of fear. Fortunately as Canadians we have constitutional rights and freedoms that allow us to choose how to take care of our bodies."

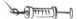

"My daughter who is now 19 months old is unvaccinated and is possibly the healthiest child I know. She is followed by a naturopath who says she is a vision of health. Do keep in mind that we better her health in every way possible (or so we think) such as feeding her organic, giving her filtered water (drinking and bath water), though she does play in dirt as it will boost her system (I did so as a kid and I'm still alive). I unlike the vaccine industry (Big Parma) don't believe that we are born to die unless we are vaccinated for every little thing out there (and let's not forget to mention take in the many many dangerous chemicals in them). She eats a mostly alkaline rainbow colored unprocessed raw diet comprised in most part of fruits and veggies though we do give her some supplements (liquid whole-food supp with no fillers, fish oil (small fish to avoid mercury as much as possible), probiotics and greens). I research everything for her and try to give her only the best.

I have researched vaccines for over 7 months for about 8 hours a day which led me through many stages: at first when my wife asked me to look into it, I pretty much told her they should be safe and effective. Secondly, I thought some of them were good, some were bad but all could be improved. Thirdly, I found many lies in plain view or somewhat hidden on actual biased pro-vaccine sites such as "Health Canada, WHO", etc. Lastly, I have come to realize that all of them are horrible (the basis of them does make sense but not everything that comes along with them, even the statistics they flaunt; a quick look at the graphs of their use and the sharp decline beforehand of said illness demonstrates their lack of usefulness and the many dangers, side-effects, resulting neurological disorders, call them what you want which are understated or deliberately altered to sell/promote and encourage the use of)

I am not here to convince anyone to do as I did or even go to the extremes I have, the bottom line is everyone has a choice, everyone should question, everyone should research. I unfortunately speak of personal experience when I say people who I know vaccinated their children in most part are close-minded, are in denial and do not research (I can't pretend to know why but have my assumptions such as guilt, refusal to admit or avoiding to find out what they did might have been the wrong thing to do!)

Again this is my own personal experience, you may have had a different one and that is perfectly ok. Do however realize that doctors push what they are told to, make money off of doing so, have incentives given to them such as trips or bonuses the more they sell or push anything "medical". They are not all evil but greed poisons many a man's soul, some of them think they are doing the right thing after years of programming. This isn't a conspiracy theory, I've spoken to many doctors, specialists, alternative practitioners in various different fields about this. Doctors are people, they are not perfect, I'm not perfect but my hunger for facts, the truth, the well-being of my family, this world and its environment have led me to uncover many conflicts of interests, many unfortunate incidents, bad history repeating itself, and propaganda. Please inform yourself, knowledge is power. If at least there is a public outcry to demand unbiased facts, investigate, conduct studies of vaccinated vs. unvaccinated children, things can only get better in my opinion."

"While my first born son suffered in the Autism Spectrum after his MMR shot, my second born daughter has enjoyed nothing but perfect health and at fourteen years old remains unvaccinated. She becomes incensed when kids just line up blindly for their shots at school, "Don't they even ask what's in them or if there are any negative effects?" My children are the only ones in their classes who deny taking the vaccines.

With regards to both my children's development, I know the difference. Not just experientially as a mother, but also as a Clinician of Heilkunst Medicine and author of three books. After four nightmarish years with my son where he was hospitalized seven times for constipation so severe he was once put under general anesthetic to have the impacted stool removed manually. There were days that he just sat in a corner, rocking back and forth like the pendulum on a clock. He also wouldn't make eye contact and his speech and growth were profoundly blocked and inhibited to the point that at 18 months I thought we might lose him in another bout of severe pneumonia. My daughter's experience was exactly the opposite.

My daughter unfolded naturally, beautifully and with ease. Not only was she not vaccinated, but she also never had the need for antibiotics or even cough syrup. By this time, I was studying and training to become a Heilkunstler. In fourteen years, I can barely count on one hand the colds or flus she's suffered. My son and daughter have been both Waldorf and home-schooled and it was clear to see that she is unfolding socially and academically with ease and joy. My son, on the other hand, suffered some major challenges requiring extra help. An example was that when he drew a tree, his roots never touched the ground! He also felt challenged by basic concepts in the early grades.

I'm thrilled to say that my son is now 17 and thriving. He has sung in the national choir, enjoys trampoline acrobatics, Parkour and Aikido. His average in the academic stream in public school where he's now integrated is 88%. He loves environmental studies and is looking to study Bowen upon graduation. My daughter is achieving similarly and she continues to unfold naturally also engaged in training as a hunter/jumper and dressage rider at the Olympic level. I'm so proud to be the mother of these gentle, loving, capable and thoughtful individuals."

Allyson McQuinn, DHHP, Diploma Homeopathy Heilkunst Program, DMH, Doctor of Medical Heilkunst, JAOH, Post Graduate Journeyman in Anthroposophical Orgonomic Physical and Medical Heilkunst, www.arcanum.ca

"In September 1991, when our son was born, we were faced with the decision to vaccinate him or not. I knew that there were problems with vaccinating children, but there wasn't much information available about why.

One of the books I read was *Confessions of a Medical Heretic* by Dr. Robert S. Mendelsohn. By the time I was finished reading Dr. Mendelsohn's book, I knew that I would be playing Russian roulette with my son's life if I were to give him vaccinations. Our doctor was not pleased but didn't hassle us.

Our son did catch whooping cough when he was a toddler. When we took him to the hospital, the nurse said that even if he had been vaccinated, it would not have protected him from that particular strain of the disease. As a young teen, he caught chicken pox, but was over that in a week.

Because our son was home schooled, he was not exposed to a lot of viruses from other children. Now he is in college, where his class mates often have colds or flus. This winter (2011-2012) he had the flu for just a couple of days and a few minor colds. He is a healthy, very physically active young man."

"My son is 10 years old and completely unvaccinated. He had an ear infection when he was about 12 months old. Within a few days he had a cough that lasted 3 months, until we brought him to a naturopath who prescribed herbs which cured the cough. At two, on purpose he caught chickenpox from his vaccinated cousin which left him mildly uncomfortable for a day. At five he woke up one day and couldn't walk or stand on his legs. He did not have any other symptoms, no fever, rash etc. and was in excellent spirits. He was diagnosed with 'toxic synovitis' which the doctor said was not uncommon and to come back if he couldn't walk in four days. Luckily we had an appointment with an 'energy' practitioner the next day who cleared his system of 'rubella'. Shortly afterwards the pain in his hips disappeared and he has had no trouble since. I do believe he 'caught' rubella from another child who had been recently vaccinated.

He is a strong, robust child who has a very healthy diet. He's gifted, conscientious and a kind person. He may have had the flu twice, a cold twice, if that. We chose not to vaccinate and it is a decision I will never regret. Being a homeopath myself, and having done a lot of research about vaccines, I felt quite confident. If only the public knew what they were really getting into by vaccinating their children."

Sandy Wright, Canada, www.wrighthealthcentre.com

"Mother of 2 unvaccinated children. The kids have traveled extensively (i.e.: to S. American and Indian farms to the Middle East, through Europe and North America)

Both kids are overall very happy and healthy. They are calm and well-behaved in the most trying of circumstances (i.e., long flights!). They are sociable and do well academically. I have resorted to conventional medical assistance for each once in their lives so far. They don't have asthma or skin issues, rarely, if ever get colds or ear pain.

In retrospect, I would have used homeoprophylaxis and other measures going through India. We were all fine until the plane back from India where I felt my stomach churn and my then 2 year old began a long episode of tummy stuff which, thankfully, has resolved with combined CoRe and Heilkunst treatment and some diet modifications.

I was recently advised by a school that my children would need to be vaccinated in order to attend and that this was solely because the children had been out of the country for more than 3 months over the past 5 years. It turns out that that information was false. I do not blame the school representatives for the misinformation. The government provided information lends itself to confusion. Upon investigation and communication with the Government, I was requested to draft and sign a further (unpublished) letter (undisclosed in any public documents according to the government officials - more than one confirmed this) to elaborate more specifically *which* vaccines my children had not had and were not to have. Another hoop to jump. The government personnel were friendly, though, which was nice. I am more thankful than ever to the Canadian Constitution which has enshrined the right not to vaccinate. Best to all parents who find themselves deliberating on this issue."

"I have 3 children ages 5, 3 & 1. My 1st was vaccinated until 18 months and the other two are completely unvaccinated. My children are very healthy, other than the occasional runny nose and cold, they are rarely sick. Never had ear infection, strep, bronchitis, or whatever other sickness kids these days. Whenever they do get a little sick, it never lasts long. They have neither allergies nor any other health condition. My first had eczema as a baby. Not my other two. They've never, not even once, have needed to take antibiotics. It seems that kids all around are often sick with ear infections, strep, or whatever else as well as many allergies, more than just to nuts.

I feel at peace with my decision not to vaccinate. After reading much on the subject, the bottom line is that I just found that vaccines (along with their producers) are untrustworthy. I prefer to trust my children's God-given bodies and a lifestyle to keep them healthy."

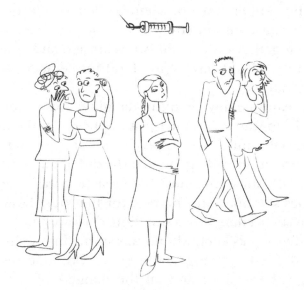

"I am a single mom of a 4 year girl. In the past I have been fully (over fully vaccinated). In 2001 I had done an archeological dig in rural Eastern Europe for 4 months through my studies at Ottawa

University. The university fully encouraged us to be vaccinated. And so, innocent as I was in the field of vaccination I made an appointment with the local travel clinic. In Canada, we have a fully financially covered medical program and of course this includes vaccinations. However, the local travel clinic was not financially covered as these vaccines go above and beyond the "regular" vaccines series. Nevertheless, they convinced me that I needed a long list of vaccines to avoid life threatening diseases. Of course at the time (early 20s) I did not know much about the issue of vaccination and never thought about researching a tiny little liquid that would be injected in my body. To no surprise, I did not see the connection to the vaccinations I had received and my sudden "allergic" reactions that are still somewhat ongoing. I developed severe reactions to scents. Anything with a scent (soap, fabric softer, hand cream, room deodorizers, perfumes etc.) and had an immediate reaction. When I would inform people of these reactions they either did not seem to believe me or they were annoyed with my constant complaining of such "smells". I finally put the two together only about two years ago and clued in …yes it took a while. Also, I have some food intolerance (sulfites and other preservatives)

In the meantime, my beautiful daughter came along. When I was about 4 months pregnant I just happened to be at the right place at the right time. I so happened to start chatting with a lady (a nurse) who started telling me that she did not have her children vaccinated. Of course my immediate reaction was "this woman is insane…does she not want the best for her kids? How could she put them in such a dangerous situations?" However, the idea stuck with me. A few weeks later, when I was sitting in my chiropractor's office, a video was playing about some USA vaccine specialist (sorry, forgot her name) and all the dangers of vaccinations. I asked to borrow the video and had a little one on one with my TV that Friday night. The info revealed was quite an eye opener for me. Afterwards, thanks to the wonderful world of the Internet I started doing some heavy research on the subject. It did not take long for my mind to be made-up when it came to vaccinating my soon to be born child. Eager to spread my great discovery, I shared my new found knowledge with friends and family. I have to say, my info was not received well. Most looked at me as if I was an alien. Even though this is only 4 years ago, it seems that there is much more awareness on the subject today then there was 4 years ago. I had to be strong and hold my end with the family doctor. With every visit she would question my motives and tried hard to change my mind. However with time, I believe she finally gave up questioning and probably views me as a "lost cause". My daughter is a tall lean toddler who is the picture of great health. I would consider us "granola eaters" in the sense that we eat very well (fruit veggies, organic meat, etc). Of course she has had the sniffles, a cold or two, stomach bug but nothing noticeable. She bounces right back from any illness. I am a teacher, exposed to germs all day long. She is exposed to germs from sick kids from her daycare and germs that stick to me from sick kids from my school. However, compared to friends of mine who have kids her age and who are constantly taking days off for their sick kids or taking them to the doctors, I am nowhere near that reality.

When she was several months old, the H1N1 scare hit the planet. People around me tried to convince me in every way possible to have her vaccinated. I even heard my own parents say that she would die and it would all be my fault. Even though I fully researched the info prior to making the decision, I adhered to my decision of keeping her vaccine free. In a short period of time following the "city mass vaccination" I noticed instant reactions to vaccines from kids in my class, family members or friends. However, no one ever wants to pin the "blame of these side effects" to vaccines.

Today, I am currently in a custody battle with my daughter's father who has decided he is now ready to be a father and "suddenly" wants joint custody of her (that I am disputing). Having very little to help his case, he has decided to dispute my choice of non-vaccination, claiming I have executed bad parenting choices and exposed my daughter to (possible) severe health issues. In Canada, not many cases like this have been to trial so it's difficult to predict where this will lead too. The outcome is to be determined...I am keeping my fingers crossed."

"Our beautiful daughter has never had any of the common illnesses of her friends, both older and younger. She has NEVER had to take any medication (which we are not opposed to if acute requirement and no immediate safer approach is viable), never had ear infections, eczema, yeast infection, throat infection or severe cold where we had to seek acute care. All of her friends we know of around the same age have had at least one (and most two) of those issues and all are vaccinated. HOWEVER, I don't believe that vaccination is the sole reason for such illnesses. I do, however, believe there is an obvious link which should NOT be ignored. Our child crawled and walked at the typical age, however, she started to speak multiple combined words at age one and progressed rapidly from that point onward. She knew all of her shapes, alphabet and numbers 1-10 by one and a half and could name and recognize them all. Well before she was 2 she spoke in full sentences and today at 2 1/2 years old she relates to 5 year old children more so than children her age in many ways.

Once again though, I DO NOT BELIEVE these differences are entirely vaccine-related. There are many, many factors including genetics of parents, healthy pregnancy, diet of child (intake of quality foods/nutrients and omega fatty acids), and the parent child relationship which contribute largely to these factors. I also believe that the evidence of this survey showing the difference in health of vaccinated and non-vaccinated children is related to the amount of knowledge of the parents regarding a healthy lifestyle. Through direct personal experience I find parents who choose not to vaccinate are also more educated regarding healthy lifestyles as indeed they have also self evaluated and studied vaccination from both sides (Allopathic/traditional medicine vs. ancient and modern holistic/natural medicine) intensely, often for years. I am NOT saying any category of people is entirely one way or the other because that is NOT true. It is my personal experience and that discussed with others, however, that this is "generally" true amongst a much larger majority of the vaccinated families vs. non-vaccinated. I find a decent portion of people explore both sides but don't spend much time looking into the risk evidence side as the vaccine industry side has so much more money and resources that they almost entirely dilute the risk evidence and are very effective at convincing them of their interests and violently opposing anything contrary. Since they have the majority the pressure to think anything different is so powerful that it literally prevents many people from researching any further. The government health agencies are also 100% supportive of the "mainstream" allopathic approach and completely discount anything otherwise. Nobody likes to feel like an outcast and many parents will subside to all of that pressure regardless of how they feel simply because they are belittled otherwise.

In a closing statement I want to say that I believe 100% that the majority of people (vaccinated or not and including all medical/health practitioners) want the absolute best option for themselves, their families and those who they care for. It CANNOT be ignored, however, that all businesses first and foremost objectives require profit FIRST (as someone in business school you absolutely learn this obvious point). That fact of life, however, must be evaluated personally to determine the extent of the profit vs. honest care relationship. It must, however, be evaluated from the top down; not by judging just the individual practitioner but the industry and its largest players and interests. That is true for all industries and practices and a lot of making such determinations falls with your natural instincts vs. any pressure you feel, you truly have to trust how you feel and how what you are told, see and hear makes you feel while remaining open minded.

The most important thing is trust and if someone, an industry, company, organization or group has been caught lying, skewing the facts or being knowingly dishonest in any way you must question their motives and evaluate how that breach of trust influences your decisions. So trust, trust yourself and your instincts and feelings first and foremost. Don't take everything for face value and most importantly don't let anyone make you feel guilty for your decisions. Trust yourself, never stop learning and always keep an open mind, not being afraid to change your decisions if trust, the evidence and your instincts point you in different direction.

Reach out to people around you and do not isolate yourself to only specific groups, remain accepting and genuinely compassionate."

"I am the mother of 3-year-old in Ontario, Canada. After much research and deliberation, I opted not to vaccinate my daughter with any of the recommended vaccinations. Thankfully, I have a fairly supportive family so I wasn't met with any resistance at all (mostly questions). My husband trusted that I did my research and that I would know best so he was also supportive. To date, we couldn't be happier about our decision.

My daughter is the healthiest, happiest, brightest little girl imaginable (and I'm not just saying that because I love her). She is leaps and bounds ahead of other children her age (her preschool teachers point this out to me almost daily). I'm grateful for this as she's a December baby headed into a JK/SK split class this September ... so she'll be the youngest by far. I have no concerns. Socially and cognitively she will not suffer at all and in fact will put some of the older kids to shame with her abilities.

In addition to not being vaccinated, she eats a predominantly organic and GMO free diet and is highly supplemented with top-quality supplements. The benefits of this combination speak for itself.

My daughter is exceptionally healthy, has no allergies, never goes to the doctor, has never been on antibiotics or had an ear infection, has a great personality and is incredibly smart. I have another child on the way and I won't change a thing ... why would I?

I feel sad that other parents haven't yet come to the same conclusions I have. I see so many sick and developmentally-challenged children and can't help but wonder if they could have been healthier if other parents were more informed about the potential risks and associated side effects of vaccinations. I tend to keep my opinions to myself, but I do feel very strongly that vaccinating our children is a mistake and not worth the risk."

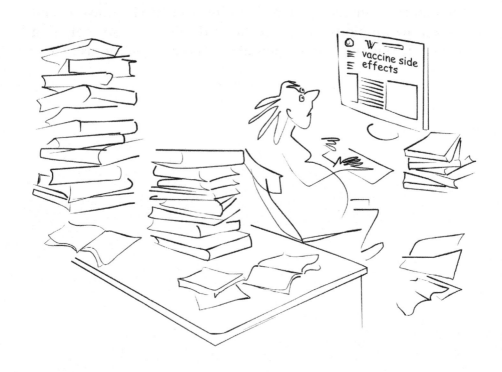

UK

"Well, my daughter (4 years old) is 100% vaccine free; she is the 3rd generation of our family who is 100% vaccine free. My grandfather had a horrible reaction to a vaccine back in the 40's and decided he would never vaccinate his own children (5 of them). So my father was unvaccinated and we (3 of us) were also unvaccinated. My father questioned everything when we were kids and decided he wasn't going to vaccinate us as it couldn't be good for a young baby to have all those chemicals injected right into their bloodstream.

I was the lucky one as I have since had the Internet for all my research. I knew I wasn't going to vax my child but I wanted to do my own research so no one could say I didn't know what I was talking about. I spent a lot of time on the subject and money. I spoke to private docs for their opinions, bought books only written by doctors and scientists. I didn't want yet someone else's opinion, I wanted the truth.

I always get complimented on how healthy, bright and intelligent my child is. She's four now and has yet to visit a doc. If I think she's unwell I take her to a homeopath (we have been twice). She has a good diet and lots of fresh air and exercise.

My unvaxed father hasn't been to the doc's for over 30 years, me for 17 years and my daughter never. As a child, I had some of the childhood illnesses such as whooping cough, chickenpox, measles, rubella, and mumps. All were quite mild but have given me lifelong immunity. My parents haven't been ill for a long, long time; they too had most of the childhood ailments, but all fine with no complications. My parents are very healthy, they are in their sixties now and last year did a coast to coast walk which was over 200 miles. They backpacked and slept in a tent for a month while on their walk. They also did another walk after that which was longer at about 240 miles. They go to the gym 3 times a week and have no health problems at all. They are also vegetarian. Myself, I'm 32 now I don't have any health issues either, I exercise 3 times a week, eat well (I'm also vegetarian and so is my daughter). We get the odd colds but nothing that requires any medication."

"I live in the UK and have a healthy and vibrant 3-year-old daughter who is, I am proud to say, completely unvaccinated. She has no health problems, no allergies, no food intolerances, and takes no medicines. She is by far the healthiest kid in our street. Is this due to her avoiding vaccines? I believe so, but as the 'powers that be' never fancy comparing the health of vaccinated and unvaccinated children in a scientific manner, I guess I can't prove it. The fact that this kind of study has never been done by manufacturers or governments says it all.

Our experience of the health authorities here in the UK wasn't too bad - I know some people get bullied a bit, but we only got a bit of gentle pressure after my daughter was born. If you know what you're talking about and stand your ground, the midwives/health visitors don't seem to push things. Our parents were harder work, the vaccine dogma seems to run deep in their generation I'm afraid.

I recall a neighbour (a pharmacist) telling me how many children had died of measles at his hospital in London. I then had to point out to him that the last child to die of an acute measles infection in the UK was in 1992!! Once you do your research, the level of ignorance surrounding vaccines is quite depressing, even amongst so-called health professionals.

Although I have strong feelings about avoiding vaccines, I almost always keep my views to myself - experience has shown me that people can get very defensive about the subject. I have absolutely no regrets about not vaccinating my child, but sometimes

I wonder how parents that have decided to vaccinate feel. Once it's done there's no going back, and even if they have doubts, I think it's virtually impossible for parents to admit to themselves that they might have done something that has harmed their children.

To parents thinking about not vaccinating their children, I would just say do your research, read widely and don't just absorb the mainstream views. You will discover that there is a lot of bad science, dirty money and dirtier politics surrounding vaccination."

"My Vaccination Journey. As a baby, I had a bad reaction to the first whooping cough vaccine. I cried most of the night and my Mum didn't put me to bed but kept me in her arms all night. I sometimes wonder if she had put me down to sleep, whether I might have been another victim of cot death. If the medical profession does not know for sure what causes cot death, how can they say without doubt that vaccines do not cause it?! As a precaution, I never received any further doses of pertussis. I went on to get whooping cough as an adult which wasn't very nice as I was caring for my 2 year old daughter who had it at the same time. Thankfully, she came through it without any problems and seemed to have a physical and developmental growth spurt afterwards.

As an adult, I fainted on two separate occasions, after having the Hepatitis A vaccine for a holiday abroad. I only fainted when I had another vaccination at the same time as the Hep. A which leads me to believe that multiple vaccines must be a bigger threat to the immune system.

However, I still believed vaccines were necessary to protect our children from harmful diseases and when my first daughter was born and was so healthy, I didn't contemplate not vaccinating her; I didn't want to take any risks.

Fortunately, the MMR controversy prompted me to do some research into single vaccines but the more I researched, the more I became concerned about all vaccines. After a lot of reading, research, soul searching and discussions with different health professionals, I came to the conclusion that vaccines possibly do not prevent the diseases they are intended to protect against and probably weaken the immune system and predispose to allergies, auto-immune disorders and other more serious conditions. As a consequence, we decided not to vaccinate any more and our second and third daughters are completely unvaccinated. I truly believe this is the best decision I could ever have made for my children. I now firmly believe that a child needs a strong immune system for optimum health and I do not see how injecting a cocktail of chemicals and unnatural substances into their bodies could help.

Our daughters are now 11, 9 and 5 and compared with other children, are very healthy. They have had their share of colds, coughs, fevers, sickness bugs and minor childhood illnesses. They have all had chicken pox and our youngest had whooping cough when she was 2 but none of them have any allergies and thankfully, cope well when they are poorly.

When our first daughter was little, she had many fevers which lasted for days and lots of colds and coughs. She was diagnosed with glue ear at the age of 4 and the hospital wanted to take out her tonsils and adenoids which I felt should be a last resort, especially as she wasn't bothered by the glue ear at all and wasn't suffering from any sore throats, ear infections or hearing loss. During the next few months, I looked closely at her diet and cut down on her dairy foods which she loved and I substituted cow's milk for goat's milk. I introduced Manuka honey into her diet and took her to a cranial osteopath who prescribed a Colostrum supplement for her. When we returned to the hospital a few months later, her glue ear had gone and she was discharged. The first doctor was adamant that it would not disappear and she would need to have her tonsils and adenoids out so I felt an immense amount of pride to realize that I had managed to prevent her from having an operation to remove an important part of her immune system and I realized that the doctor doesn't always know best! From that point onwards, her health went from strength to strength and my confidence in knowing what is best for my children also went from strength to strength!

Our second daughter seems to have the constitution of an ox and is rarely poorly. While she was little, her temperature occasionally went up while she was asleep but she would sleep through it and be fine the next day. Her colds and coughs only last a day or two but she was prone to "catching" sickness bugs! When she was 4, she damaged her front tooth and an abscess developed so the dentist decided to take it out. I then had another confrontation as he wanted her to have the tooth taken out under a general anaesthetic in hospital which again, I felt was not necessary. He then agreed to a ridiculous 3 step approach to taking her tooth out! On her first visit, she was to try out the gas; on her second visit, she was to have the gas and a needle in her gum to numb it and on her third visit, he was finally going to take her tooth out! I decided I didn't want him anywhere near my daughter and asked for another dentist. Thankfully, everything went smoothly, she avoided a general anaesthetic and her tooth was removed on the first visit without any problems at all. The only thing she remembered about the experience was a numb mouth and the toys in the waiting room! Again, the experts do not always know best!

Another decision I have wrestled with was whether or not to bring down temperatures with fever reducing medication. I now believe that a fever is a vital part of the immune response and I observe my children closely and put my trust more in the healing abilities of their bodies. Even the NICE guidelines (National Institute for Health and Clinical Excellence) state that "*antipyretic agents do not prevent febrile convulsions and should not be used specifically for this*". In 2011, the AAP (American Academy of Paediatrics) issued a new set of guidelines urging parents to avoid excessive use of fever-reducing medications when their child is running a temperature - "*Fever, however, is not the primary illness but is a physiologic mechanism that has beneficial effects in fighting infection. There is no evidence that fever itself worsens the course of an illness or that it causes long-term neurologic complications.*" However, I do believe there is a time and a place for medication and would not refuse it if I felt it was necessary.

If anybody reading this is struggling with their decision at the moment as to whether or not to vaccinate, I would urge you to do your own research; read lots, both for and against; speak to many different health professionals and then make your own mind up. An informed decision is the best decision. This time of deliberating can be quite lonely if you do not know anybody else who feels the same. Fortunately, my Mum was a big support and I subscribed to "The Informed Parent" whose newsletters gave me a regular boost of confidence that I was doing the right thing. I also started to become more interested in natural health and the immune system and I would thoroughly recommend the books by Ian Sinclair. I discovered there was an immense amount of apathy in the community so I stopped talking about vaccination and no longer felt a need to pass my opinion! I felt that my children were too precious to just "follow the herd" so I decided to inform myself which gave me the knowledge and confidence to make the best decisions for my children. I believe that striking the right balance is the answer. I try to provide my children with a healthy, balanced diet with occasional treats, lots of fresh air, sunshine, exercise and rest. I do not believe in home schooling and being obsessed with being perfect. I try to ensure my children have a balance in their lives in all areas and are able to mix in many different circles and experience all that life has to offer. I try to encourage them to follow their dreams and be happy and if some sweets or a cake make you happy from time to time then that has got to be good for you too!

Apathy, especially with regards to our children, does irritate me immensely but I also find the attitude of those who insist on controlling every aspect of their children's lives quite patronizing and over the top. None of us are perfect but we should always try to do the right thing and have the courage to keep going when difficulties arise. It is also important to say "sorry" once in a while and admit that we're not perfect!

UK

The people I am most grateful to for helping me to reach an informed decision are: Andrew Wakefield, who made me question vaccination in the first instance; Magda Taylor who runs "The Informed Parent", for providing informative newsletters and helping to give me the confidence to trust my decision and Ian Sinclair for his wonderful books and wisdom on natural health. I would also like to thank my Mum for her continuing support and my three precious little girls for providing the inspiration to me to set off on this wonderful journey!

I would like to make it clear that this is my story and my opinions, based on my research and my reasoning. I would urge you to do your own research in order to come to an informed decision. "The answers to life's questions lie inside you. All you need to do is look, listen and trust."

Mrs L Morey

"I am not anti-vaccine. I just do not believe that the huge amounts of vaccines are necessary. In the right place they can be and are an essential part of modern life. That said vaccines are not submitted to the same rigorous testing as drugs. The evidence clearly indicates that there are significant hazards associated with the use of vaccines. Some more so than others.

When my wife decided that she wanted a child we decided that we would take time to decide what we should do. We are aware that children of parents of 'mixed context' may have immune challenges, i.e. parents from one part of the world living in another. Alexandra was born of a Russian mother and British father some 7 weeks premature, just 1.9kgs.

There was no way we were going to allow her to face additional challenges other than recovering her normal body characteristics. She has been loved intensely, cherished and nagged and is nearing her 4th birthday. She has had the normal run of viral infections contracted from other children. On one occasion, with tonsillitis she required antibiotics. Strangely she eats little meat, perhaps some inherited trait from the times her mother lived in Russia.

There is no evidence of her having any rashes, allergies, etc. She is a most advanced and enquiring child for her age, a pleasurable and beautiful girl, now 1.03 meters in height (above average) and about 20 kgs (entirely normal weight range), who gets a warm reception from all who meet her. Why would we want to do anything which would place her at risk? We had a consultation and decided to get her vaccinated with several single vaccinations when the time was right i.e. when she was free from infections and her immune system was clearly at an acceptable level. Perhaps soon we will get her vaccinated against polio or tetanus or ... perhaps not."

"I have three children, one daughter and two sons, my daughter being the eldest. When my daughter was born, we had no idea that there was even a choice with regards to vaccinating our new baby, let alone any knowledge of anything else at all to do with any of the baby vaccines. We just went along with whatever a health professional recommended we do, which is what everyone else seemed to do at the time. So my daughter received the baby vaccinations, all three doses, but when it came to the MMR we learned that there was some controversy surrounding it and its possible side-effects. This prompted me to do a little research about it, and I barely touched the surface with what I could find at the time, but what I found caused my husband and I to decide that we would still like to protect our daughter from these so-called dangerous diseases so we opted for the single vaccines, at great cost to my in-laws as we weren't able to pay for them. Half way through the program of three separate shots I found out other things that made me stop in my tracks, and also fueled my desire to keep on researching and to find out as much as I could about them. I bought a few books and spent a long time on the internet, and decided that what I found was enough for me to say no to the third and final one of the three, rubella. I found I really regretted giving her any of the immunizations at all having not known anything about them before having them administered to her. I breastfed her until 7 months, and she was only fed organic and completely natural foods for the first two years of her life, I checked every food packaging label for signs of unwanted, unhealthy and unpleasant ingredients but I never did this when about to vaccinate. I have spent years dealing with the guilt and wishing I'd not done it, but have realized that you can only do the best you can with what you know at the time and so that was all I could do.

I went on to have two boys who are completely vaccine-free, and I have no intention of letting a needle near them as long as I can. They have been very healthy, one is 6 and one is 4. My 4-year-old unfortunately inherited an allergic tendency from his father who suffered terribly with eczema as a baby and child, and went on to develop asthma, so I am really glad I haven't vaccinated him for that reason, too. Apart from this he has been the healthiest of the three, rarely suffering from sickness bugs, only ever having a few short-lived colds, and a possible once a year fever lasting no more than a day or two. My 6-year-old is much the same, but my daughter who is now 9 was different as a toddler. She suffered her first bad cold at 8 months of age, she went on to be one of these children whose nose is constantly running and I felt that although she didn't get ill very frequently, when she did, she always seemed to suffer with it worse than the boys did. She is now a healthy 9-year-old and seems fairly resistant except for one or two mild illnesses a year. The boys seem to go a long time without getting anything, none of them have ever had an ear or chest infection, the boys have never had to have an antibiotic and my daughter only once for impetigo.

When I decided to stop vaccinating I began to use homoeopathy, and have done ever since. Homeopathic medicine is our first port of call for any family complaint from the very minor to the more severe. I recently used homeopathic medicine to clear up a very nasty skin infection that my 6-year-old son developed after a fall and bad graze to the knee which got infected. The nurse we saw couldn't believe we'd cleared it up with no antibiotic. So all in all I am very glad that I have kept my children mostly free from this incredibly doubtful and inconclusive method of protection from illness. I fully believe in nurturing the immune system naturally and will continue to do so. I strive to feed my children a healthy, varied and balanced diet containing plenty of fruit and vegetables. This, together with homeopathy, herbal medicine, nutritional supplements and aromatherapy essential oils forms a fantastic way of ensuring family health without unnecessary toxic chemicals which are constantly being linked to ill health later in life. Please keep up the good work encouraging vaccine-free families to share their experiences."

"I am a Doctor of Chiropractic and father to two healthy boys aged 2 years exactly and 9 months (as of March 2012). Although I am a Chiropractor I was educated at a college that provides a well balance education and I am in no way anti-medicine, my father is in fact a GP (medical doctor). After lots of research (the truth about vaccines by Richard Halvorsen, a medical doctor, being one of the most balanced reads) and soul searching, and despite attempts to persuade us and warn us of the dangers of not vaccinating by my medically orientated family and a doctor, we decided not to vaccinate our boys. I can say now how very happy we are with our decision.

Our boys are both happy and healthy in every way. They are as kids should be, full of the joys of life everyday and full of energy and enthusiasm. They have never been ill, except for mild colds which pass quickly, never had antibiotics or other medications. Compared to kids of similar age we see at toddler groups the boys stand out. And I feel very sad to think of all the stories we hear about friends´ children being so sick so often and always needed to visit their doctors, and often being filled with antibiotics or other medicines. With lovely clear skin and eyes, both seem to glow with health and wellbeing. I also believe my 2 year old to be very advanced for his age with his speaking, communication and learning, this has been confirmed by a relative who is a speech and language specialist. Of course diet and upbringing have such a large part to play in the boys' wellbeing, they eat a whole food based healthy diet without processed foods, and I certainly believe that in not vaccinating we have given them the best start in life."

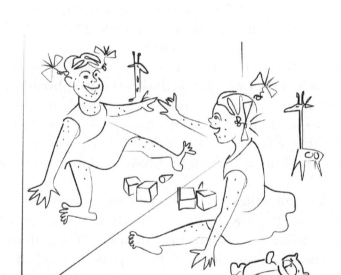

"I am the mother of 5 unvaccinated children, ages 16, 14, 12, 9 and 5. My first child was bottle fed due to doctors forcing an episiotomy on me that caused a very severe amount of pain (so much so I could not walk or sit). The site became infected, spread and nearly killed me. I was very ill for 3 weeks after her birth and by the time I was well enough to feed her, my milk was gone, so despite her being born vaginally, and me knowing I would NOT vaccinate, feed organic food, use homeopathy etc, my poor little girl was bottle fed. I was gutted. However, she was fantastically healthy despite this and did not get her first illness till 6 months of age (gastroenteritis - I believe from bottle feeding). Because she had NEVER been ill before, I panicked and rushed her to hospital. The Dr. smirked at me and asked 'Are you a first time mother, by any chance?'

She had measles at 15 months old (I believe caught from a child who'd had MMR - she sat next to him when he'd just had his MMR that day and then 2 weeks later she began with measles symptoms. 2 weeks is the incubation period for measles). She got over it quickly with only homeopathy and tepid sponging.

After that she didn't get ill again till age 2 years (she had one ear infection at 2 years and one ear infection at 3 years) - both of these ear infections I believe were caused by lack of breast milk as I later had a further four children who received breast milk after her and none of them ever had an ear infection at all and I have never had to deal with an ear infection in 14 years of parenting life, something I believe is exceptional. It isn't genetic as I had many ear infections as a child and have had weak ears my whole life.

She then got chickenpox at 4 years (something we don't vaccinate for in the UK anyway) - she didn't even get a fever or feel ill and was eating and playing like usual. The only difference I noticed was she complained of itchy spots, so chickenpox was a very mild illness in my children. Her two younger sisters had it at the same time and didn't have any trouble with it either. My fourth child had it at 4 years old too and she didn't feel ill either. Sharp contrast to me as a vaccinated child I felt really nauseated and had a fever when I had chickenpox.

After the age of 4, my eldest wasn't ill again (except for the odd cold) until she was seven, when she had a vomiting bug. She fractured her elbow jumping over a see-saw when she was eight (that was the first time she ever received a conventional pain medication).

She has not had any illness bigger than a cold since she was eight and she's now 16 and finishing her GCSE exams. She gets the occasional headache which is her biggest complaint. She very rarely catches bugs - when others get them she doesn't pick it up. When she was a baby, the health visitor remarked on this and said what a good immune system she had and this has continued into her teenage years.

My second child was strangled on her cord at birth in a botched hospital delivery and was born grey in color and not crying. She had a few more health issues I believe relating to that. She could not latch on correctly, made me bleed all the time and breastfeeding failed at 10 weeks. She was floppy, disinterested and delayed in some of her milestones and I noticed it right in the delivery room when I asked the midwife 'what's wrong with my baby?' It took 12 years to get a diagnosis of Asperger's syndrome (I believe caused by lack of oxygen during birth). We improved her co-ordination and balance and got her toilet trained by the use of a chiropractor. Apart from floppiness and delayed milestones due to Asperger's, she caught whooping cough at 10 weeks old after breastfeeding failed. She was treated homeopathically and was fine, although it did last three months. She has had no other health issues, no allergies etc. She broke her arm at age 4 and required surgery to fix it. That was her only major medical event. She is now functioning at her age level (14 years) and some of her Asperger's issues are healed (such as bladder control). She does voluntary work at a day nursery and is studying to become a nursery nurse.

My third child had chickenpox at 7 months old (first illness), a couple of bugs and a few colds. She's now 12 and has never required antibiotics, pain meds or anything else and she has never been hospitalized for anything.

My fourth child is similar - did not have any antibiotics, pain meds etc. until she was 4 years old and she required minor surgery to remove a cyst from her neck. Dr.'s asked me what her medical history was and I said 'none', when they asked about allergies to meds, I said I didn't know as she'd never had any.

My fifth child, my only boy, has never had any childhood illness or major illness in his life. He was naturally home birthed, breast fed till nearly 4 years old. He got facial eczema when I began early weaning onto solid foods at 5 months old. I cured this at 13 months old after taking dairy out of his diet and using a lavender skin cream. I have now re-introduced dairy and he has no problem with it. He had gastroenteritis at age one year and age 2 years. Apart from that, has only had the odd cold. He is now 5 years old, never had any medicines, painkillers or antibiotics in his life.

There is no asthma, nut allergy, hay fever etc in any of my 5 children despite the fact I have many inflammatory conditions (hyperacusis, vulvodynia, osteoarthritis, neuralgia, neuritis) and their father is asthmatic (he was partially vaccinated as a child). None have ever had a fit, not even from a fever. He and I always suffer with illnesses a lot more frequently and to a more severe degree than our unvaccinated children do."

Australia

"My Dad was a pharmacist back in the 1950's. After 6 years of pharmacy he decided that all the drugs that were being dispensed were not really helping people but causing more harm. He left pharmacy in New Zealand and went to the USA to become a chiropractor.

His whole life changed and so did his thoughts on health. He no longer was mechanistic in his beliefs but more vitalistic about health care.

My siblings and I were born between 1959 and 1964, my Dad and my Mum (who was a nurse) would not vaccinate us nor give us any antibiotics or painkillers. My Dad believed if we fought the small infections and pains when we were babies then our bodies would get the practice to fight the bigger infections and pains as we got older. It's interesting to note that I have the antibodies for many diseases, including German measles and malaria but I have never had the diseases.

I'm 52 this year and I've still not had a vaccination, antibiotic, pain killer or any form of prescribed or unprescribed medication. I have a perfect weight, heaps of energy, love life and can't complain about anything in my life. Yes I've had loss of loved ones but my physical and mental state has able to get me through the loss of my mother, sister, grandmother, mother in law and girlfriend within a 12 month period. I miss them but don't define my life as a result.

I have three children 22, 20 and 18 they too have never been vaccinated and have never had any antibiotics or prescribed or unprescribed medications, they are the picture of health and wellbeing, they have no allergies, ADD, ADHD, autism, asthma, or any physical or mental health issues. My two girls have menstrual cycles that are not even a hiccup in their month. They are well rounded healthy children and I thank the teaching of my Dad and the foresight of my Dad that he chose not to vaccinate or medicate us.

I am also a nutritionist and my philosophy is eating only real food. Fruit, vegetables, meat (organ as well), poultry, fish, grains, legumes, nuts, seeds, eggs, butter, good quality raw dairy as much as I can. We don't eat any packaged foods, I cook everything from scratch and believe that with my start in life, my outdoor lifestyle and having a healthy diet have all contributed to my family's health and wellbeing.

My legacy for my family is that my children understand this philosophy and will in turn bring up their children without the need for vaccinations and medications."

Cyndi O'Meara, Nutritionist, author, speaker and founder of Changing Habits www.changinghabits.com.au

"Hello my name is Bonnie, I live in Queensland Australia. I would like to firstly say that I myself am 25 and I have not had a vaccination since I was 4 and my brother who is now 22 has not had a vaccination since about 2, thank goodness my mother chose to do some researching when we were young and decided not to vaccinate us anymore. We are two very healthy adults and throughout our childhood were very rarely sick and if we were sick it was only a cold that would pass quickly. We did both get chicken pox when my brother was 4 and I was 6 and then again when my brother was 13 and I was 15 but other than that have not had any other infectious diseases. We have grown into two very healthy adults and could probably count on 1 hand the amount of times we have both been sick as adults. My two daughters 1 and 3 are also unvaccinated and have never had any vaccines at all. They are extremely healthy girls and have only had colds (only since my eldest started daycare 8 months ago). I have no doubts that my decision not to vaccinate will help continue their great health throughout their childhood and into adulthood."

"I would like to share my story of how my children have grown up unvaccinated. I have 3 children, 1st son 24 year old, 2nd son 23 yrs old, and a daughter aged 14.

My first son reacted badly to his first lot of triple antigen vaccinations. He had a high temp and was screaming. When I rang the doctor, I could pick the fear in her voice over his reaction. This made me seek further knowledge on vaccinations as well as my homeopath encouraging me to look into it a lot more. What I read really scared me and alerted me to the ongoing dangers of this chemical concoction. After treatment from the homeopath my son's health and happy personality returned.

My other 2 children never were vaccinated. Although, I did immunize them all homeopathically.

When whooping cough went around our school the only children who caught this were the vaccinated ones. Other parents were scared for my children saying that they were not vaccinated and they will get it, ironically they were the healthiest ones there.

My children have never suffered from ear infections, allergies, and only minor respiratory infections (e.g. cold). They have kept good health. I believe that the immune system needs to be supported and homeopathy has played a big part in being our first line of call for any approaching illness."

"Corey has always been a settled, happy child. He has had one illness in 5 years, a cough/cold when I vaccinated him homeopathically for whooping cough. I think it gave him a mild dose of it and that's why I decided to stop vaccinating even homeopathically. As a baby he required so little settling it was unbelievable. You fed him, changed him let him have a play and then put him to bed and he would happily go to sleep. Babysitters could not believe how easy he was to look after.

I truly believe after vaccinating my first son fully, and my second son to 6 months (stopped when he had a severe reaction) that our decision to not vaccinate Corey, our third son was one of the best decisions we have ever made. He has been the happiest and healthiest of the three boys. His immune system was allowed to function on its own and fight off all the bugs his brothers brought home from childcare, school and kindergarten. He is a healthy, robust child. Corey was born at 35 weeks and the nurses in special care advised me not to vaccinate due to being a preemie. I was surprised after having had to fight for our rights not to vaccinate previously but it proved the tide had turned since the dramas I had with not fully vaccinating Corey's older brother.

I have no doubt that Corey has been as healthy as he is because his immune system has not been compromised. Antibiotics during pregnancy and vaccinations compromised Corey's brother's digestive system and he has only now at the age of 8 experienced true good health. Corey has been able to eat anything and maintain a healthy body. He has such a strong constitution, great gross and fine motor skills and is intelligent for his age. I only wish I had not vaccinated his brothers so their immune systems had the same chance to function normally without a chemical, virus and bacteria overload. I have no doubt my children are sensitive to chemicals, preservatives and additives. It is reflected in their health and behavior every time they consume too many chemicals, preservatives and additives and I am grateful everyday of our lives that we saved at least one child from vaccination overload. I feel guilty everyday for what I put the others through, especially my 8yr old who has had a much more difficult start to life because we vaccinated him.

Since then I have had Corey get Chicken Pox (off vaccinated children in his school class). He got it sufficiently to get immunity but fought it off quickly and easily. He was only distressed about going to the doctor and I realized why - he has never had to go since he was a baby as he is always healthy!! His older brother (also not vaccinated for chicken pox) got it severely and has taken twice as long to get rid of it. This is the child who reacted severely to vaccinations as a baby and has had a compromised immune system ever since. We have passed the chicken pox onto to two of my nieces and nephews even though they are vaccinated! Why they vaccinate for chicken pox I do not know. I actually paid for my eldest child to have this vaccine when he was 18mths old; this was when I was naively uneducated about it all. He got spots at the time and got a few this time as well - have no idea whether he will get again now, where as the other two should have good immunity now."

"My story is a bit different, although my 3 year old daughter has never been vaccinated she does have ASD, I think its mild and we have chosen a treatment not supported in most countries. I have never been vaccinated myself, I chose this for both of my children. I also have a 7-month-old son who seems to be free of ASD, as he is my second child, I can clearly see that my daughter was affected from birth and probably before. She was conceived via IVF, at the time of egg retrieval, my husband had a high fever, a urologist suggested a procedure where they collect sperm that had not been affected by the fever, they develop the sperm in the lab and perform ICSI. My better judgment was screaming NO but the medical team assured me this would be fine. At age 2.4, my daughter was diagnosed with ASD. We feel very good about our choice to not vaccinate her, had we done so I believe she would have been much much worse. My son was not conceived the same way and he is so much different than my daughter at this age. We chose to do stem cell therapy with my daughter. I know autism is brain damage or missing healthy cells in the brain and throughout the body, in choosing stem cell we are actively regrowing and replacing damaged and missing cells. It is still early only 5 months post stem cell, but we have had enormous improvement. Still a long way to go but we are getting there rather quickly. Dr. Rader from Medra has had 100% success rate with this therapy and there are patient histories where children recover fully from ASD, so we are hopeful our daughter will only keep getting better.

She had a little speech up until age 2 then lost it all, woke up one morning and just said dadadadada. It was the scariest time on my life. She is getting her baby babble back and even starting to say words now.

I took an online course from Sheri Nakken on the dangers of vaccines prior to having children, so I know the dangers and know how vaccines contribute to autism. We refused everything at the hospital with both my kids, no Vit. K, no eye goop and I had delayed cord clamping with my son even though he was an emergency C section.

I feel very good about my choice, we only practice homeopathy. I don't even take my son to the doctor for well visits, he is very healthy, and apart from the ASD my daughter only gets colds.

Update: 7 months post stem cell therapy for my daughter. On the anniversary of my daughters 6 months post stem cell, we had another child psychology evaluation, we had moved to Australia from San Francisco. We noticed the difference in Amelia three weeks ago, she was starting to talk, single words, asking for things, and was immensely interested in children, in playing with toys, was very eager to explore outside her comfort zone and was extremely happy. She was a very different child, it feels like she is returning to the little girl she was at age 1.5 when it seemed she was free of autism. The evaluations were very different this time, she was diagnosed with late development and on the fence of the Autism Spectrum Disorder. The psychologist was asking what we had done to get such fast results. The first evaluation at age 2.4 she was spinning, looking outside the side of her eyes, she did not smile for 1 year, did not want to reach out to her dad or anyone, she was poo smearing, was running away from social situations, wanted nothing to do with children, was avoiding eye contact. We could not take her anywhere without a giant meltdown. This evaluation she looks you straight in the eye and even stares, approaches children and plays alongside children, wants to play with them but is still not sure how. She is not doing any of the weird ASD behaviors, she is the happiest little thing I've met, always smiling and laughing and dancing. Dr. Rader tells us the two stem cell therapies four months apart, will replace or rebuild the damaged cells in her brain. As the months and years pass she will only keep improving."

"My story is a credit to God, who put me in the company of other parents who had decided not to vaccinate. I had had all my vaccinations and had never heard that vaccinations could have damaging effects. I started to research more when I began work at a Special Needs School. Many of the students where on the Autistic Spectrum, and went through terrible times at regular schools as well as in our smaller independent school, due to their heightened sensitivities and social disabilities. Soon I began to consider that even the slightest risk of incurring Autism was too high a risk for me to take. Instead I improved my diet and health through pregnancy, and persevered through breast-feeding as long as possible for my two sons (11 months). I researched healthy eating from their first solids, and have avoided all chemical additives, sugar, gluten, and processed foods as much as possible in their diets. They are now 5 and 7 and have never had an ear infection while their little toddler friends had countless ear infections and many ended up having surgery to insert grommets. They have both only ever vomited on two occasions in their whole lives. One has had antibiotics for strep throat, but the younger has never had antibiotics. The younger has had a bit of croup, but I treated it successfully with homeopathic preparations. They still catch a cold or get a fever, but it never seems to last as long as it does with the kids they caught it from. They are clever, happy and energetic – so energetic that my husband often teases me that I should feed them junk food to slow them down!"

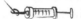

New Zealand

"We have 3 children, Saskia 25, Tamara 22 and Oliver 19. Saskia only had the first 6 week vaccination. After that my neighbor gave me pamphlets by Hillary Butler from NZ, on the dangers of vaccines and I quickly realized what side effects these vaccines could have for my child. After reading a lot of material including the book, "A shot in the dark", I was not going to let any doctor inject my children with some vaccine that I had no idea what contents it had and how my children would react to it. I also realized that it was my job to be responsible for their health, which meant I controlled what they ate. So not much junk food, mainly food that was made at home and often grown at home too. In the last 25 years we had no need for a family doctor. We did use a naturopath a couple of times. Once when Tamara was about 4 months old for Craniosacral massage, as she cried a lot. And after one visit she was fine. And once for Oliver when he was 18 as he had suspected scurvy from working and eating at McDonalds.

As you can see our children are now adults and they have to make their own decisions. What I am glad about is that they have learned that whatever you put in your mouth will affect your health. And although they are far away from perfect they know immediately what to do when they don't feel well. Just adding to eating right I do have to stress that the food today is not the food that I grew up with. The nutrition level has decreased incredibly low because of the farming methods and all the environmental impacts on the land e.g. pesticides, polluted water, polluted air ... In addition we take organic supplements to boost our immune system on a daily basis. And I just want to add one more observation (two of our kids still live with us, so lots to observe). If we don't supplement, our immune system very quickly deteriorates and we feel unwell. Luckily, we know straight away what to do."

"After lots of research into the pros and cons of vaccinating, we decided that for our family and for our baby the benefits of not vaccinating outweighed the benefits of vaccinating. That was before our baby was even born. By the time she was born, it was a no brainer. She was not getting vaccinated.

Her story is not long. In fact it is quite simple! She is only 20 months old now but she has been a wonderful child ever since she was born - of course with the usual ups and downs. She has not had any of the major illnesses that vaccinations are supposed to prevent but not only that, her health is better than I could have ever imagined. Her immune system seems wonderful - alongside healthy eating, being breastfed and being well nurtured, we actually contribute the strength of her immune system to the fact that she *wasn't* vaccinated. She has not had any severe colds, flus or stomach bugs, and those that she has had, had minor symptoms that have passed reasonably quickly. She has never been 'under the weather' for more than 24 hours. Further to that she has never suffered from colic-like symptoms, rashes or any other 'baby-related' health issues. She had the chicken pox when she was about 15 months old and whilst the spots seemed severe, her other symptoms didn't last more than 24 hours (runny nose, fever, tired, low energy). Her immune system could handle it.

Of course, I have no idea if she still would have been this way had we actually had vaccinated her. I do however have myself to compare her to and other children her age who were vaccinated. I was vaccinated as a child and have had eczema, cradle cap, asthma and earaches my entire life, along with other illnesses and severe symptoms. Again, that may have nothing to do with my vaccinations but if these things were to 'run in the family' as many doctors have told me they do - my daughter has not had any of these symptoms. Further, she has had fewer and less severe colds than other children her age who were vaccinated, she is much more aware than them, she is much more cognitively developed than them, she is much more coordinated than them, she seems healthier and more comfortable than them, she has no allergies or intolerances (in comparison, every other vaccinated child I know has some kind of allergy or intolerance) and her skin and general appearance has more of a glow and brightness to it than theirs.

Again, this may all just be coincidence. You could also accuse me of being biased (although it is not just those who love my daughter that have made these observations), but regardless of what you put it down to, I would never risk vaccinating any of my children based on my own experiences and what I've seen in my own daughter and in other children."

"We stopped vaccinating our kids after our second daughter started having central sleep apnoeas which increased after each of the first three vaccinations.

Our 3rd daughter, Renata, was the one who at nine was diagnosed with a combination of Asperger´s (mild), ODD, ADD, anxiety, and Dyspraxia. Once she was finally diagnosed (I knew something was different when she was a toddler, but it took years for us to get a diagnosis), and I started reading up on it, I finally, for the first time in my life understood my father. He is very much classic Asperger´s. Way more than my daughter is. Over the years I have noticed the traits in many members of my family, and am pretty sure that a few have undiagnosed Asperger´s.

My nephew also has strong autistic tendencies, the most obvious in the extended family (6 children and 15 grandchildren), and he had a severe reaction with his first vaccinations, and was hospitalized with 'A-Typical Measles' a few days after his 4th vaccination.

My personal belief is that my nephew is more severely affected due to his vaccinations. He has not been diagnosed, as my sister does not want to label him. He is home schooled after some fairly big problems in school. Sadly, my sister has continued with vaccinating her younger child.

Obviously, there is a family history of autistic tendencies. My concern is that it can be made worse with vaccination. Not all vaccinated kids end up on the autistic spectrum, but those with a pre-determined make-up are clearly at much greater risk of developing such problems. Just like not all children have apnoeas after vaccinations. There is some sort of family problem there too, with my 6th daughter having them too - but never as many or for as long as my vaccinated daughter had them.

Sadly, with the help of the propaganda spread in university, my now 20 year old, has decided we should not have stopped giving her the shots and has started getting them. But that is her choice.

I certainly hope my now 18 year old with Asperger´s doesn't go down that route."

"Our fully vaccinated 1st born, now 18, has Asperger´s. Our 4 and 6 year olds - both unvaccinated, show signs of mild Asperger´s, but nowhere near the extreme behavior and heart-wrenching problems their older brother goes through. I have no proof that the vaccinations accelerated an underlying genetic predisposition, but looking at these three boys there is an obvious difference, and my mother-heart is very grateful and blessed that I had more information and support from friends as our later children were born. We have 6 children now - 2 vaccinated, the next had only one shot - her 6 week old shot which I was very unsure about and waited till she was 6 months old. Immediately on having the shot I felt like it was the wrong thing to do, and have felt VERY confident not to vaccinate the following 3 children."

Norway

"I'll be happy to tell the story of my unvaccinated child. He is now almost 8 years old. I am very happy to say his health is very good. In fact he has never used any antibiotics nor any other medicines. He has been to the doctor twice - once with ear infection that was caused by a virus and cleared away the next day. And once with acute laryngitis.

During the years from 1 to 6 he was in kindergarten - he was only sick (common cold and varicella) about 15-20 days altogether. The last two years in school he was not sick at all.

He never had any skin problem or runny nose. He doesn't have any allergies or reaction to foods."

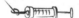

Iceland

"I am a mother of 3 children. My oldest born in 1999 is fully vaccinated, my daughter born in 2005 is partially vaccinated and my youngest born in 2010 has not received any vaccinations at all.

I was never completely at ease when it came to making a decision about vaccinating our older children and just went with "*what was usually done*" as I didn't have any credible information at the time to support a decision not to vaccinate.

It was through my studies as a homeopath that I experienced a different approach to health and found the means to do further research into vaccinations and the possible consequences.

The difference in the level of my children's health is clear and in hindsight – my oldest (fully vaccinated) may have experienced adverse reactions from his vaccinations, having to deal with delayed language development, ADD, stomach upsets, food intolerances, persistent low grade fever and regular headaches (migraine).

My second child (partially vaccinated) experienced repeated ear infections in her first year of life, which were successfully helped with homeopathy, as well as not receiving any more vaccinations beyond her first year.

My youngest and the healthiest of the lot, has never had any vaccinations. She is a very vital, healthy and happy child and in her young life she has only ever experienced the occasional cold and runny nose that blow over in a matter of days. She is often the only child at the child minder not to fall ill with the flu, get the stomach bug or have a bad cold.

I am very happy with our decision not to vaccinate and I have never doubted the decision. I only wish I would have had the resources to do the research into vaccinations earlier, so that all of my children could enjoy a strong and healthy natural immunity."

Poland

"My daughter turned 3 in March. She is a totally vaccine-free kid. What I'm observing as she grows up is that from the very beginning she was very active, very reactive and 'delicate'- I mean, it was hard to calm her down or to put her to sleep. But on the other hand, she displayed all the abilities (like walking, speaking etc.) very early. Now you can speak with her about almost everything and from time to time she amazes us with sentences like: 'When you speed up, you slow the time down'.

She was born after complicated labor (finished after 12h with cc), very small (2,8kg) and only 6 points Apgar. But she did not get newborns jaundice and after 24h observation, when I got her, she was one of the healthiest kids in hospital. To me that's important - we're from Poland and here newborns are given two shots during the first day: BCG and hepatitis. I strongly believe that there is a link between strong, prolonged jaundice of newborns (very, very common among Polish babies) and that hepatitis shot.

She was breastfed until she was 1.5 years of age (until 0.5 year - only breastfed). And since she was 1.5 she went to daycare.

I find her very healthy- she has minor allergy problems, the same I have: we both don't tolerate milk and cats. But she has never been given antibiotics in her whole life. No lung infections, no bronchitis, no ear infections.... A year ago she got chicken pox. It took 6 days from when we saw the first spots until she went back to daycare. No fever, not so many spots, very mild. Few weeks ago she "passed something on" to me and my husband, probably some Rota infection. We were ill for a whole week. And she had almost no signs, just one evening a small fever and minor intestinal problems. Next day- healthy kid! And we were struggling SOOO

HARD! During 'running nose season' she gets common colds from time to time (2-3 times/year), but it's always just 2-3 days and she's healthy again.

So, in conclusion, I'm very happy we made this decision. I'm sure 'from inside', that it was absolutely right."

Netherlands

"The only thing that is a little bit concerning is their moderate alcohol-abuse as students (with the three of them). Hopefully this will disappear as life becomes steady and serious.

Their health is perfect, apart from catching a cold once a year (by loss of healthy immune system or stress-induced). No allergies, no eczema, no bronchitis, no ear-infections.

My eldest daughter (35 years) has swimmer-eczema (candida). My second daughter (26 years) had once a herpes infection and sometimes a cold. My sons (24 and 22) are sportsmen and they only have injuries resulting from their activities.

The sons endured the mumps two years ago. The youngest one with the complication orchitis at one side. It was very painful and he was not amused, but no bad words about our decisions. In their environment there were more students, vaccinated, who got the mumps-infection.

In their childhood they got rubella, scarlatina, measles, whooping-cough, varicella twice, and three-day fever. They sometimes missed school because of a cold or a throat-infection. Never for long and they never got antibiotics, antipyretics, or other regular medicines. Never been in a hospital, my son once only for a wound. They all have been in tropical countries (no-yellow-fever-areas) and never took vaccinations. They took homeopathic remedies with them for prevention and cure.

I'm very content with our choice for natural circumstances in development, without disturbances by vaccines. In our family we use preferably homeopathic and anthroposophical medicine. The choice of my children for their own babies is in their hands."

Germany

"My children and I have all not been vaccinated, and that is because the midwife who took care of me during my pregnancy made me aware of the fact that after the birth of my child I would be confronted with a range of preventive medical interventions and that we should get the information beforehand so that we would have a position in the matter and could reject it if we thought it was necessary. Her own position was critical, except for vaccinations where she was wishy-washy. For example she said that she used to recommend to people to not have the "U4" vaccination, and that she had been reprimanded for doing that [by her superiors] and that was the reason why she was no longer able to dissuade people from having that vaccination. So I was sort of confused and said: "So then we shouldn't have it?" and she shrugged her shoulders. I asked her what was so bad about it, and she rolled her eyes and whispered that it was terrible and that 30% of all children that she took care of had to be treated for early symptoms for diseases such as neurodermatitis (dry cheeks).

I tried to do some research. In the internet I only came up with advertisements until I entered "vaccination" and "damage". And the text with the subtitle "We live in hell and everybody is watching" by Buchwald opened my eyes. And when I looked at other people in my family, the less the parents had vaccinations done and the later the healthier the children were. What a coincidence. There are three severe side effects that we have that I know of. One of my sisters almost went blind when she reached young adulthood. I myself had to deal with a life-threatening auto-immune disease on my kidneys after I was vaccinated. And a cousin of mine had a particularly bad time with MMR, he experienced a regression of his language abilities and all sorts of other things that are associated with that. The marriage fell apart on account of it, his father was hit by a car after having had too much alcohol; his mother occasionally has alcoholic binges, and the sister and the mother agree that children ruin your quality of life and that it would be better not to put any children into the world at all.

So I say, no, not children, but vaccinations. But she continues to think they are the thing to do because the disability could have just as well have occurred after the measles. She herself works with handicapped children as a nurse and so I guess she is sort of ignorant in that respect.

At any rate, my three children are the picture of health and can develop and unfold freely without their bodies having to cope with these serious poisons. I don't think I would be able to live very well with not knowing what kind of unknown damage a vaccination could have on my child. So at least I warned my sisters and my cousin, who had the bad luck of being married to a man who came from a family that traditionally was very much in favor of vaccinations. She was able to postpone the vaccination, but because her son wears glasses and somehow is somewhat delayed in his developments, is prone to bronchitis and things like that, I think that her husband – who is now her ex-husband – asserted himself."

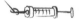

"My husband and I are both doctors and until the birth of our first child we never really looked into the subject of vaccinations. We simply had all the vaccinations that are recommended done because that is how things were done. But when our daughter arrived I suddenly started remembering unpleasant experiences that I had had as a child myself in terms of vaccinations. I wanted to save my daughter from having similar experiences and started to look into the basics and scientific proof that have to do with vaccinations in detail. Unfortunately my own academic studies did not help much. There you learn the same about vaccinations as you do when you read standard package inserts. First I wanted to find out what vaccinations are really necessary and which were not, so that I could spare her them. My list of vaccinations that are necessary quickly became shorter and ultimately I realized that no vaccination is really necessary.

At the same time I realized that the idea of vaccinations and all of the propaganda that accompanies it is rubbish and the assertion that life is saved, etc. etc. In the meantime, we have three children who have not been vaccinated at all. All of them were born at home, were breast-fed for a long time and have grown without medical interventions. They are healthy, they are ahead of their peers in terms of development and they are a joy for their parents. When they get sick they usually have a fever for one night and the next day they are fine again. We adults are sometimes jealous of that. For me it is normal to have healthy children so that I do not contemplate that very often. But when I see other families I know that it is not normal. In the mean time I have become skeptical of all kinds of medicine. Not vaccinating is only one aspect that is important to me; there is also a healthy life style and healthy food. Then the body becomes resistant and robust in a natural way and does not all kinds of palliatives products, homeopathic globuli, medication and vaccination in order to remain healthy or to get healthy again. Finding out what kind of food is really healthy is another subject that is not easy. When the conditions are really good, diseases that occur are not matters of life and death that one has to be afraid of but rather they are processed by a healthy immune system, as planned. I have learned that and am now not afraid of diseases, but I am willing to learn how one can achieve natural health under these optimal conditions."

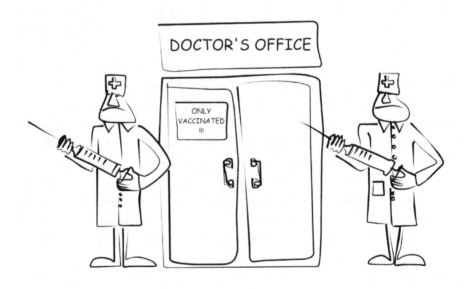

United Arab Emirates

"I have a partially vaccinated son, now 5 years and a completely unvaccinated daughter, 3 years. I had very strong feelings against vaccines already with my first pregnancy and was strongly decided not to vaccinate at all. Unfortunately, I had a very uncooperative pediatrician, who kept scaring me and disregarding all my concerns. It was a very tough time and I feel with every parent going through that phase. Now I would just go to another doctor. But then I had my first baby, so small and helpless and I eventually gave up. So my son got DTP and polio, starting at 3 months, in divided doses very far apart. Thank God he never had any reaction and I hope that this is partly because he was a fully breastfed baby and his immune system had time to wake up a little before the first vaccine "insults". He never got any vaccines after those.

I was continuing doing my research on vaccines and got more confident and now I can easily argue with any health care professional. I got many books and DVDs which I give to each pregnant friend of mine to help them make their decision.

With my second baby, I also had a peaceful natural birth (although in hospital), delayed cord clamping, no vaccines, no drops, no separation of mother and baby. I feel very strongly about the first hour after birth and bonding. I was lucky to find a new pediatrician who respects my choice not to vaccinate.

Having sort of tried both approaches I can easily compare the health of my children. My son as a baby had more colds, coughs and had to take antibiotics twice so far in his life. But I strongly believe his immune system is strong and has overcome the vaccine's harm, as he was breastfed for almost 2 years and I am a nutritionist so I dare to say we eat pretty healthy all the time.

My little girl loves doctors! Because she never has to go to any! She only used to go for checkups and had once a cold, otherwise she is incredibly healthy and resilient little girl. She never had a cough syrup, Panadol or antibiotics. Thanks God.

Being surrounded by super vaccinated children, the difference in their health is obvious. My children almost never miss school because of sickness, usually 1 or 2 days per year. Almost all other children have allergies, asthma, learning problems and very common colds."

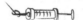

Indonesia

"I am a mother of a healthy 13 month son. After I gave birth I never go to the pediatrician because, thank God, my son is always healthy. The most serious illness he ever suffered from was a 3 days common cold.

I live in Jakarta, the capital city of Indonesia, where vaccination is obligated for children. But I'm not alone, many parents choose not to vaccinate their children, and thank God, all of their children are healthy and seldom go to doctor."

India

"I have two daughters, both unvaccinated. The older one, Kyra was born on Oct 3, 2008. She has never had to take off from play school/ school due to health reasons. When I enrolled her in play school at 2.9 years, people told me that she was going to start falling sick frequently due to association with other small kids but thankfully she sailed through her time at play school. She has traveled with me to sea and sailed with her father for months together without any concerns away from any doctors.

She has been on homeopathy since birth, but unfortunately, she was given a vitamin K shot without our knowledge soon after she was born...Kyra has had atopic dermatitis since she was 2 months old. While most of it is resolved with homeopathy, some bit of it is still remaining on her arms. Other than the skin problem, which remains on the surface, she hasn't had any health concerns... barring a few cold and cough episodes that would have lasted not more than 2 days...or just some reaction to something bad she has eaten which resolves within an hour or so with homeopathy. My younger daughter, Inaya is almost 6 months old and hasn't taken any vaccinations either. She has stayed in perfect health and hasn't had any time where I have needed any doctor support. Also, wanted to mention how Kyra, compared to almost all kids her age displays far more energy all through the day. She travels 45 minutes to school and comes back active, not needing any nap at home either..."

Appendix

Survey on the state of health of unvaccinated children

December 29th 2010 the German website www.impfschaden.info and the English counterpart www.vaccineinjury.info started to conduct a survey on the state of health of unvaccinated children. Due to social network pages and the help of many people who supported the survey and placed links on different webpages, currently as many as **15000** questionnaires were filled in.

The results presented here are not a formal study but rather an informal piece of personal research. Nevertheless the results of the survey were compared with the results of the German study KIGGS. The KIGGS study was designed as a comprehensive, nation-wide, representative interview and examination survey for the age group 0-17 years. Between May 2003 and May 2006 a total of 17,641 participants were enrolled. The data obtained from each study subject included objective measures of physical and mental health as well as parent- or self-reported information regarding the subjective health status, health behavior, health care utilization, social and migrant status, living conditions, and environmental determinants of health. Although the KIGGS study and our survey are not 100% comparable they show huge differences in common illnesses.

Most participants on vaccineinjury.info came from the USA, followed by UK, Canada and Australia. The graphic below shows the distribution of the different countries.

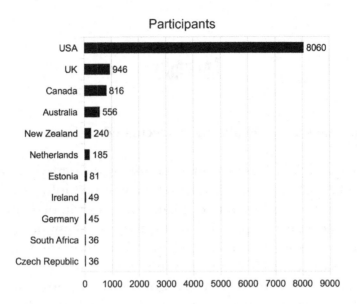

Gender and age distribution

The gender distribution is very balanced with slightly more male participants. Most participants were in the age group 0-2 years, followed by 3-4 and 5-6.

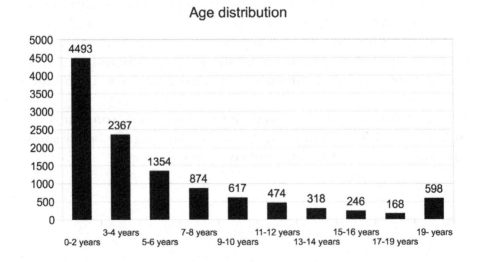

Appendix

Preferred treatment
The parents stated that their preferred treatment was naturopathic and homeopathic health car services. Only 8 % said they preferred conventional medicine. Treatment in the "other" column was mainly chiropractic and supplemental.

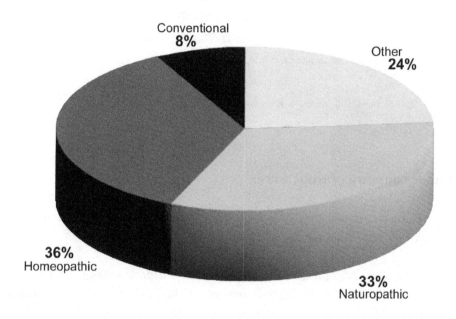

Reasons for not vaccinating
The reasons given for not vaccinating were mostly that the parents had concerns about the ingredients in the vaccines and were of the opinion that vaccines are not effective. More than 50% stated that they are afraid of side effects. 25% said that they had

a vaccine-caused injury or vaccine reaction within the family or friends and decided not to vaccinate anymore.

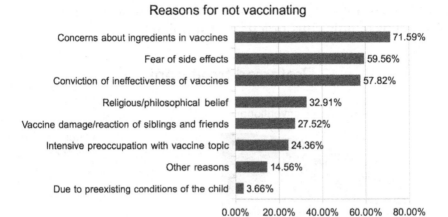

Other common reasons were:

"Concerns about the lack of long term studies of the effects of vaccines. Also a lack of studies on the effect of multiple vaccines."

"As a speech-language pathologist in the pediatric setting, I have seen many cases of children having seizures within 36-72 hours following routine vaccines with a traumatic regression in the child's brain and language and overall development. I feel in my heart, it is linked to vaccines and do not want to subject any of my children to this."

"The belief that not enough is known about the establishment of the immune system and its development. Concern that intervening with vaccines at such a young age could be creating problems in the immune system. Essentially the risks of vaccinating infants are mostly unknown at this time."

"Because I want him to build natural immunity"

"Too much, too soon for his developing mind and body. I want to give him time to develop, rather than bombard his system"

Appendix

"I feel that not vaccinating my child is my choice, not the govts. I think it's crazy that everyone constantly tells me how he will not be able to go to school if he is not vaccinated, I guess as always, ignorance is bliss. I am well educated and I have a college degree, so I have to do extensive research on the pros and cons to vaccinate or not to. It is not just a light decision that I made over night!"

"Lack of long term safety studies, lack of full disclosure/obscuring truths about vaccines, their efficacy and side effects, safety and testing."

"To make a stand and say I will not put things into my child that has yet to be proven without a doubt to be safe."

"He is exclusively breastfed– he gets all of the immunities from me that he could possibly need. A lot of these "vaccine preventable diseases" aren't even all that serious, we are just led to believe that they are because of course, doctors and pharmaceuticals make bank from administering vaccines!"

"I believe "it's the soil, not the seed." Raise healthy people and disease will be a thing of the past."

"There are no head to head clinical trials comparing vaccinated vs. unvaccinated children and their comparative outcomes. Why do all other drugs go through such testing, some with a control group, and vaccines don't? His 2 brothers have some vaccines, but I stopped once I began doing my own research/literature reviews. Having determined that the body of data in support of vaccines is weak and the overall lack of quality control studies has led me to this decision. In the past, prior to children, I was in the pharmaceutical industry and am well aware of the types of studies that need to be conducted prior to drug approval. I am very saddened that the vaccines are not held up to higher standards."

"Anti government control. Can't have raw milk? OMG! We are forced to get shots? I will die fighting this! I am a true American and I have freedoms and I will fight for them!"

"I have an evolutionary approach to child rearing. I trust 4 million years of evolution more than a generation of experimentation on something as complex as the human immune system."

Illnesses in unvaccinated children

The results of our survey show that unvaccinated children are far less affected by common diseases than vaccinated children. The following chart shows the comparison between our survey and the KIGGS and other studies.

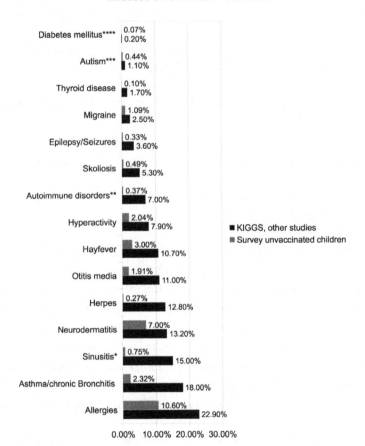

Illnesses unvaccinated-vaccinated

* http://thorax.bmj.com/content/55/suppl_2/S20.full.pdf
** National Institutes of Health
***Jon Baio, Prevalence of Autism Spectrum Disorders — Autism and Developmental Disabilities Monitoring Network, 14 Sites, United States, 2008, March 30, 2012 / 61(SS03);1-19
****National Diabetes Fact Sheet

It seems that the vaccination status of the parents plays an important role in the development of certain diseases in their children. The parents who reported autoimmune diseases in their own children were asked in a follow up study whether they themselves were vaccinated as children or later in life. There was not one parent who was unvaccinated and had a child with an autoimmune disease. This is probably valid not only for autoimmune diseases, but for other common illnesses such as asthma, autism, neurodermatitis, allergy, hay fever, herpes etc. where the immune system and genetics play such critical roles in the lives and health of children. From this, I believe, we can surmise that these illnesses become worse with each vaccinated generation and the progressive assault on the genetics and immune systems of all those involved.

For more detailed analyses please go to http://www.vaccineinjury.info/survey.html. You can find analyses subdivided into different age groups, analyses of the influence of breastfeeding and different treatment options.

New Children Book!

Sarah doesn't want to be vaccinated

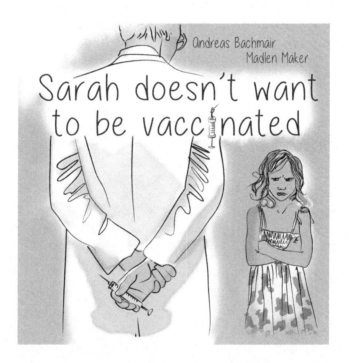

Sarah is really excited about the upcoming Girl Scout trip but there is a problem: she has no vaccination record and doesn't want to be vaccinated. Can she still go or will she have to stay home?

This book is dedicated to all children and parents who are concerned about vaccinations and refuse to give in to the constant vaccination propaganda. Parents who refuse to vaccinate their children make this decision after careful consideration, because they are convinced that vaccinations do more harm than good. The decision not to vaccinate is often not an easy one, because one so often faces criticism and seems to be swimming upstream.

Dear parents, I hope this book will help you and your children to understand better the controversial issue of vaccination.

The book is available in American and British English, Spanish (Sara no quiere vacunarse), German (Sarah will nicht geimpft werden), Italian (Sara non vuole essere vaccinata), French (Sarah ne veut pas être vaccinée), Dutch (Sarah wil niet worden ingeënt), Russian (Сара не хочет делать прививку) and Danish (Sarah vil ikke vaccineres).